INTERMITTENT FASTING FOR WOMEN OVER 50

THE BEST WAY TO RESET YOUR METABOLISM AND DELAY AGING

HOW TO QUICKLY LOSE WEIGHT AND BOOST YOUR ENERGY IN A HEALTHY WAY

(21-DAY MEAL PLAN INCLUDED)

D1715276

LOUISA PER

First Printing Edition, 2021

Printed in the United States of America

PERFECTBOUND2.0

Available from Amazon.com and other retail outlets

Published by Perfect Bound 2.0 Design and Writing © 2021 Perfect Bound 2.0

Table of Content

Introduction

When it comes to losing weight, women over 50 often have a difficult time. This may be caused by a variety of factors. Poor metabolism, aches and pains in joints, a loss of muscular mass, and sleep deprivation are the most common. You do not have the physique of a young person anymore. There are meals that may no longer suit you and activities that may cause you difficulty. And it is at this time that illnesses such as cancer, heart attacks, metabolic diseases, and diabetes are most likely to develop. After you become 50, intermittent fasting (IF) is a wonderful way to reclaim your youth. IF's anti-aging benefits help you remain youthful and avoid a variety of age-related illnesses.

What is intermittent fasting (IF)?

IF refers to conscious control of the amount of time spent without eating. It may be done for a number of reasons, including convenience, lifestyle choices, health, and weight reduction. Intermittent fasting poses two fundamental questions:

- How long did it take you to eat your final bite one day and your first meal the next?

- Would you be willing to prolong that time frame? How frequently do you do it, and by how much?

Your responses will form your understanding of intermittent fasting, which most likely change over time as you will gain self-awareness and experience. Most forms of intermittent fasting do not tell you what you can and cannot eat; instead, you are forced to think about time while planning your meals for the day.

Furthermore, it is probably a good idea to clarify what intermittent fasting is not. IF is not a green light to eat anything our eyes see as long as you 'starve' yourself for the requisite amount of time. Anyone who approaches intermittent fasting from this perspective is doing more damage than good. Because you are organizing the intervals at which you eat, the foundations of excellent nutrition, lean proteins, lots of fruits and vegetables, excellent sources of fiber, and excellent fats, do not alter. Maintaining excellent nutrition with the periodic reward is essential if you want to get all of the advantages of intermittent fasting.

The concept of IF has nothing to do with deprivation. The phrase "starvation" suggests that you do not have food and are suffering from the consequences of not eating. In most cases, starvation is not planned or premeditated. Intermittent fasting, on the other hand, means that you have access to food but may choose when to take it, and the process is not as harmful to your health as starving would be.

Keep in mind that intermittent fasting is not for everyone. It is not something that everyone should do. It is merely an approach that may be beneficial to certain people.

Once you have decided to try intermittent fasting, keep in mind that you will need to eat healthily as well. It is unreasonable to expect to lose weight and boost your health by overeating at mealtimes.

Why does it work?

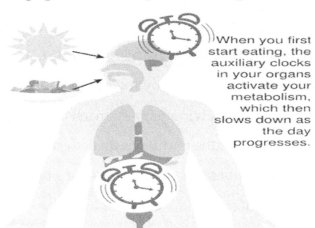

Your body's natural clocks
Your brain's master clock wakes you up with morning light and makes you tired at night.

When you first start eating, the auxiliary clocks in your organs activate your metabolism, which then slows down as the day progresses.

Intermittent fasting includes consuming calories mostly during the hours of the day when your body is most capable of handling them.

It may seem too easy to be successful, but intermittent fasting benefits because it enables you to operate with your body's natural metabolic cycle by setting a clear distinction between eating and fasting. The human body was created to be productive during the day and sleep at night. The internal clock that enables you to maintain this wake/sleep pattern on track is called circadian rhythm, and it is stored in your brain and is triggered by light. However, there are auxiliary clocks in your organs that are triggered by your food consumption. When you eat, your digestive clocks are activated, and they get to work, assisting you in effectively digesting, absorbing, releasing, and storing energy. The clocks in these vital organs, on the other hand, wind down as the day goes on.

As a consequence, meals ingested early in the day are processed more effectively than those ingested subsequently in the day. You may work with your body's normal cycle to become a more effective metabolic machine by lowering the number of hours you eat. You will be giving your stomach a break during your fast, which will reset the hormones that affect your weight. This time of rest also liberates up resources for your body to clean up and heal itself.

It all leads back to hormones, your body's messengers, whose signals direct your organs what to do. Hormones are created while your stomach is busy digesting food to help you utilize the energy from that meal. Hormones play a significant role in storing surplus energy in locations like adipose (fat) tissue if you eat more than you need right now. This is how body fat accumulates.

Chapter 1: The History and Myths of Fasting

Quick, constant access to food is a relatively recent idea in the history of civilization. People had to depend completely on the land for their nourishment prior to the Industrial Revolution. They could not just get in the car and go to the local food shop if they were hungry. Hunted and collected as much as they could throughout ancient civilizations. Food, on the other hand, was not always certain. The shooters and gatherers would return with a new corpse and a bunch of fruit and berries on certain days, but they would return empty-handed on others, particularly during times of shortage, such as the winter months. They were effectively fasting on these days, even if they were not doing it on purpose. These fasts may last days, weeks, or even months, depending on the time of year and the ability of the hunters and gatherers.

1.1. The Origin of Fasting

Fasting has been recommended for spiritual growth and health enhancement since ancient times. Fasting only as religious tradition arose independently among people and faiths all across the globe. Fasting was thought to boost cognitive ability and attention by the ancient Greeks. *"The finest of all remedies is resting and fasting,"* stated Benjamin Franklin, one of America's founding fathers and the alleged creator of the lightning rod and bifocal spectacles. Fasting is typically defined as cleaning or purifying process when utilized for religious reasons, but the essential premise remains the same: refrain from dining for a predetermined length of time.

Spiritual fasting, contrary to medical fasting (which is intended to cure sickness), is considered a crucial catalyst for whole-body wellbeing, and a broad range of faiths believe that fasting has the capacity to heal.

Fasting is a technique for **Christians** to clean their souls so that their bodies are pure, and they can connect with God. Lent, the forty-day season between Ash Wednesday and Easter, is one of the most popular seasons for Christians to fast. Those who observed Lent in the past decided to give up food or drink; now, Christians may still refrain from food or drink, but they frequently opt to go without a particular item. This custom is intended to commemorate Jesus Christ's forty days in the desert, during which he was obliged to fast.

Fast Sunday is a **Mormon** ritual in which members refrain from eating two meals (for a duration of 24 hours) on the very first Sunday of each month. In an additional effort to clean and purify, members share personal experiences with their church group during this fast. They also contribute the equivalent of those two meals to the church in order to help the poor; a process called a fast offering.

Fasting is said to enhance spirituality in **Hinduism** by denying the body's physical necessities. Although fasting is a normal aspect of Hinduism and is practiced on a frequent basis, Maha-Shivaratri, or the "Great Night of Shiva," is one of the most widely observed fasts. Devotees fast, take ceremonial baths, worship in a temple, and practice the values of integrity, forgiveness, and self-discipline during Maha-Shivaratri.

Fasting is a technique for **Buddhist** monks to exercise control from relying on human cravings, which they think is a key to obtaining nirvana. Many Buddhists fast every day, eating breakfast but not eating again until the following morning. Furthermore, Buddhists often fast for long periods on just water.

There are various reasons to fast in **Judaism**, including seeking God's compassion, commemorating significant life events, expressing appreciation to God, or grieving; nevertheless, if you are fasting alone, it is customary to keep the fast secret.

Ramadan, yet the most popular religious fast, is a **Muslim** tradition. During Ramadan, Muslims refrain from eating and drinking from dusk to dawn, as well as smoking, sexual intercourse, and any other potentially immoral behaviors.

Fasting—and the slight dehydration that results from a lack of fluids—is said to purify the spirit of harmful impurities, allowing the heart to be turned toward spirituality rather than worldly cravings.

There were just a couple of the faiths that use fasting as part of their devotion. Pentecostalism, Sikhism, Catholicism, Taoism, Baha'i, Jainism, Anglicanism, Methodism, and Lutheranism are among the faiths that practice fasting.

1.2. What is Medical Fasting?

Fasting was first used as a medical treatment for some of Hippocrates' ailing patients in the fifth century B.C.E., earning him the title "the father of medicine." "To eat while you are unwell is to nourish your sickness," Hippocrates said in one of his famous statements. He felt that fasting enabled the body to concentrate on treating itself and that pushing food into a sick condition may be harmful to a person's health since, instead of focusing on healing, the body would spend all its energy on digesting. When ill people did not eat, their digestive systems would close down, and their bodies would focus on natural recovery.

1.3. Facts and Myths on Fasting

The fact is that there has not been much human study done on it, but as its popularity grows, more studies should be conducted to learn more about what it can do for health. Let us take a moment to review what we already know based on previous studies.

- **Fact: Insulin levels fall when HGH levels rise**

When you fast, your blood insulin levels decrease dramatically, making it easier for a person to burn fat. It may also increase your amounts of human growth hormone by 3-14 percent, which is an excellent fat-burning and muscle-building combination!

- **Myth: You will lose weight if you fast**

You will not see much development no matter how long you fast; if you break your fast (and that is why the very first meal of the day is called breakfast) by eating burgers, fries, and slices of pizza, you will not see much development. Once the fast is over, you must continue to eat consciously. You are cancelling out whatever advantages your body receives from fasting if you regard each feasting time as a cheat day. To lose weight, you must still maintain a calorie deficit in your diet.

- **Fact: Intermittent fasting has been shown to reduce inflammation**

Intermittent fasting may really reduce inflammation in your body, which may be a tremendous lifelong health benefit, protecting you from developing arthritis, GERD, and sometimes even allergies. This is not show-stopping information to remember while you perform your bicep curls, and it may make a big difference in your health's durability.

- **Myth: When it comes to weight loss, fasting is superior to snacking during the day**

Several studies have shown that IF almost nothing has to do with long-term weight reduction. It does not matter whether you consume those calories all day or only during a 4- to 8-hour window to lose weight; the key is to maintain a continuous calorie deficit.

- **Fact: Fasting is good for your heart**

Different techniques of intermittent fasting have been demonstrated in certain studies to lower blood pressure, enhance insulin sensitivity, enhance heart rate variability, and lower cholesterol, all of which reduce the risk of cardiovascular disease and stroke.

- **Myth: Fasting makes you more stressed**

Short-term fasting causes little stress to the body and has no effect on cortisol levels, the stress hormone. Fasting, in fact, may protect overall cortisol levels low, which controls your immune system, keeps your blood pressure in check, and helps your body burn fats.

- **Fact: Fasting may help your skin clean up**

Your system is able to concentrate on other restorative processes when you pause from eating. This permits the body to eliminate toxins and control the operation of other organs, such as the kidneys and liver, which may help your skin clear up.

- **Myth: When you fast, your body goes into hunger mode**

Your body will consume energy in a variety of ways, but it will not starve. The human body is built and adapted to withstand fasting for brief periods of time. Furthermore, there have been studies that suggest fasting may have health advantages.

- **Fact: Fasting has been shown to benefit long-term brain health**

Fasting boosts neuronal health by increasing the synthesis of a specific protein brain-derived neurotrophic factor (BDNF). This potent protein may safeguard your brain cells against the neurological abnormalities that come with Parkinson's and Alzheimer's disease.

- **Myth: Fasting makes it hard to concentrate**

There is no evidence to suggest that IF has a damaging impact on cognitive processes. Short durations of fasting, whether for Ramadan or for medical purposes, have been shown to increase cognitive performance, boosting quicker learning and memory.

Chapter 2: Why is Fasting Actually Good for Over 50 Women's Health?

Lean muscle mass, a slower metabolism, difficulties resting, irregular periods or menopause, and joint discomfort are among difficulties that women over 50 faces. This has a significant impact on their quality of life. IF is a nonpharmacological strategy used by several medical disciplines for a wide range of disorders from ancient times to address these concerns. Women, on the other hand, benefit from a lighter approach to fasting since their hormone production and activity differ from that of males.

Many health advantages for women are described below, ranging from weight reduction to general wellbeing to mental health:

- Weight loss

- Improve heart health

- Improve mental health

- Lower the risk of diabetes

- Reduce body inflammation and oxidative stress

- Prevent some cancers

- Cell regeneration, longevity, and immunity

- Autophagy

- Polycystic ovarian syndrome connection with intermittent fasting (PCOS)

- Cellular repair

- Skin health

- Improve muscle health

- Boost your metabolic rate

• **Weight Loss**

There are several reasons why IF aids weight loss. The first will apply to general health and fitness concerns. The second case pertains to ladies above the age of fifty. It has to do with weight gain after menopause.

In general, many ladies engage in intermittent fasting in order to reduce weight. This is the first benefit since intermittent fasting results in fewer meals being consumed than previously. This will also help you to consume fewer calories. Many of the hormones have a role in fat burning, which is greatly aided by intermittent fasting. Human fat is naturally digested and absorbed via a natural mechanism. The metabolism boosts fat burning even more. Intermittent fasting is, therefore, a direct cause of weight reduction.

However, there is a condition that commonly affects women over the age of 50. When a woman's menstrual cycle comes to an end, she enters menopause. Menopause usually happens when a woman reaches the age of fifty and has gone 12 months without the menstrual cycle. The average age of women who are afflicted by it is in their 40s, although it may also be in their 50s. It is a biological process that occurs naturally. However, it is not a simple procedure. Physical signs and symptoms are extremely prevalent. The most frequent physical symptom is hot flashes. This might potentially be affecting your sleepiness by disrupting your sleep. It is not a pleasant position, particularly for a professional woman in her fifties. Even if you are a stay-at-home mom, this might cause issues. Your total energy level will drop. Aside from that, emotional difficulties are typical among women going through menopause. There are a variety of therapies available to address the challenges that arise as a result of this natural process. Intermittent fasting is one of the most beneficial treatments for menopause.

Menopause is usually accompanied by the following symptoms:

- o Weight gain and a slowed metabolism

- o Sweats at night

- o Hot flashes

- o Periods that are irregular

- o Mood swings

- o Problems with sleep

- o Dryness of the Vaginal

- o Dry skin and thinning hair

- o the fullness of the breasts is lost

One of the prevalent issues after menopause is gaining weight unexpectedly. Why would anything like that happen? This occurs as a result of the slowing of the metabolism during menopause. This might result in unanticipated weight gain as a result of this normal biological process. This may also be accompanied by reduced insulin sensitivity, which may cause problems with sugar and carbohydrate digestion. All of this contributes to weight gain. Some women may get depressed as a result of it. Your body is beginning to behave strangely, and you have no idea how to manage it. There are ways to make the procedure go more smoothly. I have personally experienced the advantages of chamomile tea. Menopause's weight increase may lead to worry and melancholy. Intermittent fasting can undoubtedly assist you in achieving your weight reduction goals. It is a procedure that will take time and effort, but you will reap the advantages in the end.

• Improve Heart Health

Fasting regularly and having a healthier heart might be linked to how your body handles cholesterol and sugar. Low-density lipoprotein, or "bad" cholesterol, may be reduced by intermittent fasting. Fasting is also thought to help your body digest sugar more efficiently. This may reduce your risk of gaining weight and help you manage diabetes, both of which are risk factors for heart disease.

• Improve mental health

Mental capacity deteriorates throughout time and with increasing age. The body's normal cycles must be updated after you reach the age of fifty. A few women do it with the help of medicines or supplements. Nonetheless, such medications have their own set of adverse effects. Intermittent fasting increases the activity of a cerebral hormone that helps to alleviate sadness and promote mental wellness.

• Lower the risk of diabetes

Intermittent fasting, like continuous calorie restriction, seems to reduce some of the diabetes risk factors. It does this mostly by lowering insulin levels and decreasing insulin resistance.

- ## Reduce Body Inflammation and Oxidative Stress

Intermittent fasting reduces inflammation, which may lead to illnesses such as diabetes and inflammatory diseases. Several studies have shown how cell oxidative pressure has a significant influence on our aging rate. The imbalance of free radicals and cell reinforcements inside the body causes oxidative pressure. Free radicals may destroy cells, proteins, and DNA, and they are created by both external and internal metabolic processes.

- ## Prevent Some Cancers

Though the research is still in its infancy, intermittent fasting (extended overnight fasting) may have advantages for at least some cancer patients. Healthy cells are regarded to be considerably better at adjusting to their surroundings with fewer nutrients. Cancer cells, on the other hand, continue to proliferate and hence have a higher nutritional need. This might make cancer cells more prone to DNA damage and stress during medication, such as chemotherapy, and hence more vulnerable to the treatment.

Cancer prevention agents, which are compounds that are supplied by the body and may be found in a variety of foods, aid in the destruction of free radicals harmful effects.

Researchers and experts believe that limiting free radicals and increasing cancer-prevention agent contents in the body (thus lowering oxidative pressure) may help slow down the aging process.

• Cell Regeneration, Longevity, and Immunity

Cells undergo a diverse pressure response during fasting, which might indicate its multiple beneficial effects. Fasting on alternate days improves indicators of oxidative pressure and extends life span. This food restriction also activates autophagy, a cell-observation system that improves immunity.

Humans may live longer and have fewer age-related health issues, such as metabolic diseases, by following time-restricted eating habits.

• Autophagy

Autophagy is a vital procedure in which the cells of the body "clean away" any unneeded or damaged segments. Fasting and calorie restriction impose strain on the body's cells. When a person limits the quantity of food they consume, their cells get fewer calories than they require to function properly.

When this happens, the cells should be able to perform even more efficiently. Autophagy causes the body's cells to clean out and reuse any useless or damaged components as a result of the pressure provided by fasting or calorie restriction.

• Polycystic Ovarian Syndrome Connection with Intermittent Fasting (PCOS)

Intermittent fasting, or not eating for particular periods of time, has been shown to help with the symptoms of PCOS that have developed in certain women. This kind of diet reduces irritability, improves insulin and glucose levels, and leads to a significant increase in testosterone levels and ovarian capability. Fasting has also been proposed as a way to amplify the impact of testosterone overstock on the human body by limiting the amount of insulin produced, which is partially responsible for the unexpected appearance of androgens.

You may expect weight loss or, at the very least, no weight gain if your glucose and insulin levels are normal. You should also notice a reduction in chin hair development and skin improvements as your testosterone levels drop. As a result, ladies will stop waxing their faces.

• Cellular repair

Our bodies accumulate waste proteins that have no use over a period of time. Intermittent fasting triggers a process known as autophagy, which causes cells to break down. The cell divides and eliminates any by-products and proteins that are no longer needed. As a result, the body becomes cleaner. This cleaning cycle clears the way for fresh cells to be generated. At fifty or more years old, the ability to create fresh cells without the necessity for any prescriptions or supplements is a blessing.

- **Skin Health**

Diet has a significant impact on the beauty and firmness of our skin, the body's largest organ. Inflammatory diseases may wreak havoc on the body, and their symptoms range from mild to severe. Dermatitis and skin outbreaks are two common inflammatory conditions. These two inflammatory illnesses may generate unsightly markings, and you do not have to be a certain age to have them; they may even occur much later in life. Many people grow timid and withdraw from the public view as a result of these markings.

The stomach and the body are inextricably linked. Certain meals might make you feel irritated all over your body. It seems that a calorie-controlled diet plan, such as intermittent fasting, which is rich in healthy food choices and low in sugar, may assist people with these disorders to maintain or even prevent them. It is critical to ensure that you are consuming the optimum sources of food for your welfare while fasting, taking into consideration all your health requirements.

- **Improve Muscle Health**

Intermittent fasting has also been shown to boost the muscular and joint health of women over the age of 50, according to research. A part of the researchers discovered that fasting affects how the body manufactures chemicals. This will strengthen the bones and help avoid ligament issues and lower back discomfort.

- **Boost Your Metabolic Rate**

According to experts, being fasting causes a surge of the hormone norepinephrine. This hormone burns fat by increasing your basal metabolic rate. Furthermore, once you reach your calorie intake, your digestive system remains at a high level. When you consume, you are burning an excessive amount of fat!

Chapter 3: Master the Most Effective Fasting Method

Intermittent fasting includes a variety of forms. All IF approaches are effective and important but finding out which one works best for you is up to you. The following are the most well-known:

- 16:8 Method

- 5:2 Diet

- 12:12 Method

- 14:10 Method (Lean-Gains)

- 20:4 Method (The warrior diet)

- Eat, Stop, Eat (24 hours)

- Alternate Day Fasting (ADF)

- Extended Fasting

- Spontaneous Meal Skipping

- Fasting-Mimicking

- Meal Skipping

3.1. 16:8 Method

It is at this point when the magic begins! Your sugar and insulin levels are lower after 16 hours of fasting, and part of your reserve glycogen has been depleted, so your body is searching for fuel. Your adipose (fat) tissue, on the other hand, has enough energy to spare. This time without meals also frees up resources for regeneration and repair by allowing your body to rest from the energy-intensive work of digestion.

- **Instructions**

Although you may fast for any 16 hours, many individuals find that ending with supper and then missing breakfast the following day is the most convenient way to perform a 16:8 fast.

If you are going to miss breakfast, it is a good idea to consider how you will spend your early hours. It is ok to drink coffee, tea, or water. A little cream with your tea or coffee may help curb hunger and make your morning more enjoyable but be cautious of "calorie creep." The cream is mostly made up of fat. Dietary fat does not really prevent fat burning since it does not elevate blood glucose or insulin levels. The fat calories in the cream, on the other hand, offer your body a readily available energy source, forcing your body to stop using body fat until the calories are depleted. Your calories are going up to a level that suits your body's energy demands if you consume 3 cups of coffee in the day and add cream to each cup.

Fasting helps you lose weight because it deprives your body of simple energy, forcing it to rely on harder-to-access body fat. It is also worth mentioning that taking any calories while you fast may disrupt autophagy and other healing processes, so if you want to employ fasting for health advantages as well as weight reduction, avoid the add-ins and sip your coffee or tea black for the best effects.

- **Advantages**

16:8 fasting satisfies the three E's (easy to do, enjoyable, and effective). Many individuals find it simple to skip breakfast since hunger is generally lower in the morning, and the activities associated with this time of day keep their thoughts from thinking about food. Dinner may be enjoyed as a family activity. Fasting for 16 hours is also beneficial to one's health and weight reduction.

- **Disadvantages**

Fasting from evening until breakfast the following day demands avoiding after-dinner beverages and snacks, as well as reducing or eliminating coffee creamer. These lifestyle changes might be difficult.

3.2. The 5:2 Diet

The 5:2 Diet is based on the principle of fasting for two days a week. Dr. Michael Mosley developed this variation on alternate-day fasting, which is sometimes known as The Fast Diet. The plan entails calorie restriction for two days during the week and eating properly for the other five days.

- **Instructions**

The days you fast are up to you while following this procedure, although these should not be consecutive. So, you may fast on Mondays and Thursdays, but not Mondays and Tuesdays. You are permitted to eat 500 calories on the fasting days, corresponding to the modified form of alternate day fasting, with some reports claiming that males might take 600 calories. Those calories from the fasting day might be taken in one meal or spread out across many smaller meals.

The 5:2 Diet, like other kinds of alternate day fasting, is helpful for weight reduction. This effect might be due to the fact that calories are naturally lower throughout the week. 2 groups of overweight women were compared in 6-month research. One group was assigned to a standard low-calorie diet, which reduced their daily caloric consumption by 25%. The second group followed a 5:2 diet plan, which included severely reducing calories on two days of the week and eating properly on the other five days. Despite their diverse eating practices, the two groups consumed almost the same amount of calories and essential nutrients at the conclusion of the trial. This finding suggests that, contrary to popular belief, alternate-day fasting does not really lead to binge eating.

- **Advantages**

Unlike other kinds of alternate day fasting, the 5:2 approach restricts calories just on two days of the week rather than every other day. Even though effort is still necessary, this approach is the least restrictive and hence the most accessible for people interested in alternate-day fasting.

- **Disadvantages**

You may have adverse effects such as irritation, hunger, or problems sleeping, as with any high-calorie restriction. Furthermore, for some individuals, five days of "regular" eating might be a steep slope in relation to food decisions. It is natural to want to treat oneself after a hard day's work, which may translate into consuming more unhealthy food than usual on non-fasting days.

3.3. 12:12 Method

This is an excellent place to start if you are new to fasting. Consider it an overnight fast, similar to what you would do before a blood test. If your doctor has scheduled a blood test for the following morning, he or she may instruct you to quit eating after supper and not eat again until the morning of the test. It does not get much easier than that to keep a 12-hour fast.

- **Instructions**

Your day is cut in half if you do a 12:12 fast. You will eat the whole of your calorie intake in a 12-hour window and then fast for the next 12 hours. The goal of this strategy is to become used to fasting. You may learn about IF and guess it sounds fantastic, however when it finally happens to put it into practice, worries arise:

- o Will I be starving? Will I get ill?

- o Will fasting induce me to binge for the rest of the day?

When you first start intermittent fasting, it is natural to be nervous. Beginning with a 12:12 fasting can help you to overcome your concerns and gain confidence.

If you add the hours, you sleep when fasting, it becomes much easier. Begin by eating dinner as you usually would. You will not have to eat an additional portion of food to get you through the night; you will be fine. Take note of when you last ate — this is the beginning of your fast. Before going to bed, sip some water or tea, but do not eat or drink anything caloric. (Try cleaning and brushing your teeth if you are having difficulties preventing late-night eating.) Your tongue will feel clean and fresh, which can help you resist appetites and help you think twice about putting additional food in it.) After 12 hours, you may have your regular breakfast to break your fast. You have done it! Just one thing left is to keep track of how you are feeling.

- **Advantages**

You may eat three or even more meals as you usually would throughout the day as long as you limit your calorie consumption to a 12-hour timeframe.

Disadvantages

While this relatively brief time without eating may assist balance sugar levels and maintain weight, the overall weight reduction and health advantages of IF will not be fulfilled by this approach.

3.4. 14:10 Method

The lean-gains approach has various distinct versions on the internet, but its popularity comes from the idea that it helps lose fat while rapidly converting it to muscle. Through the hard practice of fasting, eating well, and exercising, you will be able to convert all that fat into muscle with the lean-gains approach.

This strategy involves fasting for 14–16 hours and then eating and exercising for the remainder 10 or 8 hours of the day. This approach, unlike the crescendo, involves regular fasting and eating rather than alternating days of eating and not eating. As a result, you do not have to be so careful about increasing your physical effort to work out on days while you are fasting since those days are every day!

- **Instructions**

Start with a 14-hour fast and work your way up to 16 if you feel at ease but remember to drink plenty of water and avoid using extra energy on activity! Remember that intermittent fasting allows you to improve your health and potential. You do not want to risk losing some of this growth by hastening the process.

3.5. 20:4 Method (The Warrior Diet)

It is debatable if the advantages of a 20-hour fast are significantly better than those of a 16-hour fast. Fasting in the 20:4 ratio, on the other hand, has piqued the curiosity of many people who want to accelerate their growth. Ori Hofmekler, a fitness specialist, promoted this fasting plan. The Warrior Diet was called after Hofmekler's inspiration: ancient warrior tribes that ate little portions of full, unprocessed meals throughout the day and one huge meal in the evening.

The classic Warrior Diet recommended a specific eating plan that included big, drawn-out evening meal rich in protein, unrefined carbs, and healthy fats. Many individuals nowadays consider fasting for 20 hours as a technique to drive their bodies to a greater degree of fat burning and cellular regeneration, despite the fact that little research has been conducted to back up these claims.

- **Instructions**

You must consume all your daily calories during a 4-hour diet plan to complete a 20:4 fast. Those calories may be taken in any manner that suits your lifestyle but having two meals between 2 and 6 p.m. is one option.

There is something alluring regarding fasting for Twenty hours, but it's not for everyone. During the eating window, the classic Warrior Diet emphasized the significance of eating full, unprocessed foods. Because clean, nutrient-dense meals were the only meals accessible, it is simple to understand how ancient warriors may have benefited from this method. We now live in a world where calorie-dense, nutrient-poor foods abound. Without careful preparation, it may be simple to overindulge in fast food and processed snacks, lowering the strategy's health benefits. As a result, you may want to consider longer fasts like this one as a once-in-a-while technique for speeding up your progression or breaking through a weight-loss plateau.

- **Advantages**

Those with a slow metabolism may notice that fasting for 20 hours is all their body needs to lose weight. It might also be claimed that the extra hours of low blood glucose and insulin levels might help those with diabetes.

- **Disadvantages**

If you start this strategy too soon, you may develop hunger and cravings, which may result in binge eating. If you view a 20:4 fast as an advanced skill level to practice once you have been comfortable with 16:8 fasting, you will have the best results.

3.6. One Meal a Day (OMAD)

The abbreviation OMAD refers to "one meal a day." Because that meal is usually eaten in an hour, OMAD may also be regarded as a 23-hour fast or 23:1 fasting. The most stringent kind of time-restricted eating is this method.

- **Instructions**

The notion of eating just once a day is simple to understand. The meal may take up to an hour and is considered a substantial meal with no calorie or macronutrient restrictions. However, bingeing on processed, refined carbohydrates is not recommended. However, it is difficult to consume enough calories to fulfill your body's requirements while eating healthful, complete meals. This result might be seen in either a favorable or bad way. Restrict nutrient intake to one meal per day has a good effect in that it naturally produces a calorie deficit, which promotes weight reduction. However, if you have too many low-calorie days in a row, your metabolic rate will drop, making long-term weight loss difficult. This unfavorable result was notably proven in a study of Biggest Loser contestants who had metabolic repercussions that lasted years after the program finished. Contestants substantially reduced their calorie intake and boosted their calorie expenditure via activity throughout the competition. Weight loss was quick due to the continuous calorie restriction. Unfortunately, this resulted in their metabolisms slowing to a level that corresponded to their calorie limitation. Their bodies responded to the new low-calorie level by burning fewer calories, making it extremely simple for them to recover the weight they had lost.

We can only hypothesize about the advantages and hazards since research on time-restricted eating seldom captures a real one-meal-a-day practice that requires consuming all calories inside a 1-hour eating window. Given the lack of evidence and worries regarding long-term calorie reduction, eating one meal a day should be seen as a strategy to throw your metabolism for a loop and prevent it from getting static rather than a daily habit.

- **Advantages**

Including an OMAD fast in your weekly schedule may assist you in breaking through a weight-loss plateau. If you are traveling or have a very hectic day ahead of you, OMAD makes life easier by minimizing the time spent preparing and consuming meals.

- **Disadvantages**

When you limit your calorie intake to one hour per day, it is difficult to receive most of the vitamins and calories you need to keep your metabolism from slowing down. If you use this strategy on a regular basis, you will get the best results if you keep track of your body fat % to ensure that you are shedding fat rather than muscle.

3.7. Fasting Mimicking Diet

Dr. Valter Longo, an Italian scientist and researcher, developed the Fasting Mimicking Diet. He wanted to recreate the advantages of fasting while also supplying nourishment to the body. His changes eliminate the calorie shortage that comes with other kinds of fasting.

The Fasting Mimicking regimen is based on extensive research and clinical investigations. Dr. Longo promotes the ProLon Fasting Mimicking Diet, a five-day weight reduction regimen based on the concepts of fast mimicking, via L-Nutra, a nutrition technology firm he founded.

- **Instructions**

Five-day prepared meal kits are included in the ProLon Fasting Mimicking Diet regimen. All the snacks and meals are made using natural foods and are plant-based. The meal packages are low in carbohydrates and protein but abundant in healthy fats such as olives and flax. Dieters eat the contents of the meal kit solely over the five-day period.

The Diet delivers roughly 1,090 kcal on day one (10 percent protein, 56 percent fat, 34 percent carbohydrate), but only 725 kcal on days two through five (9 percent protein, 44 percent fat, 47 percent carbs). After glycogen reserves are exhausted, your body generates energy from non - carbohydrate sources due to the low-calorie, high-fat, and low-carbohydrate composition of the meals. Gluconeogenesis is the name for this process.

The Diet is meant to give 34–54 percent of typical calorie consumption, according to one research. The body's physiological reaction to conventional fasting procedures, including such cell regeneration, reduced inflammation, and fat reduction, is mimicked by this calorie restriction.

Before beginning the five-day fast, ProLon advises dieters to speak with a medical expert, such as a doctor or certified dietitian. The ProLon five-day cleanse is not just a one-time cleansing; it should be repeated between one to six months for best benefits.

- **Advantages**

ProLon users have experienced increased energy, mental alertness, and focus, in addition to weight loss. Fewer food cravings and improved eating habits, the capacity to be more conscious during meals, greater drive to embrace a healthy lifestyle, a clearer understanding of food proportioning, and a greater capacity to resist sugar foods are all stated advantages participants have experienced after leaving the program.

- **Disadvantages**

You may suffer side effects such as a minor headache, tiredness, and trouble focusing when using ProLon. In addition, unlike other diets that focus on lifestyle improvements, ProLon is only intended to be utilized for a limited time. ProLon is not the diet plan for you if you are seeking something you can stick to long-term.

3.8. Eat Stop Eat (24 hours)

Eat Stop Eat is a novel method of intermittent fasting in which a maximum of 2 non-consecutive fasting days is included each week. Brad Pilon, writer of the famous and appropriately named book "Eat Stop Eat," created it. The Eat Stop Eat technique is not your usual weight-reduction plan, according to Pilon. Instead, it is an opportunity to reconsider what you have been taught about mealtime and frequency, as well as how it connects to your health.

- **Instructions**

The Eat Stop Eat regimen is pretty simple to implement. Simply select 1 or 2 non-consecutive days each week when you will not eat — or fast — for the whole 24-hour period. You may eat as much as you like the other 5-6 days of the week, but it's encouraged that you make prudent food choices and don't consume more than your body requires.

When you use the Eat Stop Eat approach, you can still take something on every single day of the week, which may seem illogical if you are fasting between 9 a.m. Tuesday to 9 a.m. Wednesday, for example, you will consume something before 9 a.m. Tuesday. On Wednesday, after 9 a.m., you will have your next meal. This ensures that you fast for the whole 24hrs — but no longer. Make sure that regular water is recommended even on Eat Stop Eat fasting days. The ideal option is to drink lots of water, but you can also drink calorie-free drinks.

- **Advantages**

It is easier to adopt, and there is no need to track calories.

- **Disadvantages**

Dehydration, hunger, and vitamin shortages are all risks.

3.9. Alternate-Day Fasting

Alternate-day fasts are done by switching between fasting and non-fasting days, as the name implies. Full and modified are the two types of versions. Every other day, you must entirely refrain from caloric food and drink in order to complete an alternate day fast. On fasting days, the modified approach permits you to ingest roughly 500 calories.

- **Instructions**

When you do a complete alternate-day fast, you do not eat anything on the days you are fasting. You could, for example, complete your meal on Monday, go without meals on Tuesday, and afterward eat again on Wednesday. Noncaloric beverages such as water, tea, and coffee may be consumed throughout the fasting time. Eat till you are satisfied within the eating window.

Dr. Krista Varady is a world-renowned expert in alternate-day fasting. She discovered that permitting the ingestion of 20 to 25% of your body's energy requirement on fasting days improves adherence without compromising the health and weight-loss advantages. On fasting days, you may eat your 500 calories in one meal or as a small dinner plus snacks. Non-fasting days are considered feasting days, which means you may eat until your appetite is satisfied.

On non-fasting days, there are no restrictions on calorie consumption or meal choices with any version. Although studies demonstrate that those who alternate-day fasted ate more on non-fasting days than they did on fasting days, the extra calories they ingested were not enough to compensate for the calories they lost on fasting days. As a result, the weight reduction reported with alternate-day fasting is attributed in part to the natural reduction in calorie consumption over time.

- **Advantages**

Alternate-day fasting is the most researched fasting strategy, with both variations demonstrating good health and weight-loss effects. Many individuals find that an alternate-day fasting habit is easier to keep than more standard diets that limit calories every day.

- **Disadvantages**

It is likely that going without meals for more than a day, as in the full version, will result in muscle mass loss. Both kinds need self-control, and hunger may arise on fasting days. Please keep in mind that the studies on this and other kinds of alternate-day fasting were conducted over a period of several months, so commitment may be required to reap the full advantages.

3.10. Extended Fasting

The idea of an extended or lengthy fast differs depending on who you ask. It is a fast that lasts more than a day. Long-term fasting has possible advantages, such as weight reduction, increased autophagy, and continuously controlled sugar levels and insulin levels, but it also has hazards. The hazards include but are not limited to muscle loss and a decrease in metabolic rate. If you are thinking of fasting for more than a day, examine the dangers and benefits and talk to your doctor beforehand.

- **Instructions**

Because prolonged fasts run longer than one day, they may easily incorporate one or even more nights of sleep, resulting in fasts lasting 36, 48, or even more hours.

- o **36-hour fast**: You may fast for 36 hours by stopping eating at 7 p.m. on day 1, skipping every meal on day 2, and afterward eating again at 7 a.m. on day 3.

- o **48-hour fast**: You may fast for 48 hours by stopping eating at 7 p.m. on day 1, skipping every meal on day 2, and then eating again at 7 p.m. on day 3.

- o **Multiple-day fasts**: Such fasts require going without food for many days in a row. There is no specific length of time to fast, though 3 – 7 days is a common range.

Except for a 36-hour fast, which is similar to the complete alternate-day fast, long fasts are usually spread out and done on a monthly basis rather than weekly. Nothing except water is consumed during a real long fast. Noncaloric beverages or carbonated fluids might help you get through the fast while also potentially providing health advantages. Salt and other essential minerals may be lost during lengthy fasts; thus, carbonated liquids might help.

When you go for a few days without eating, your digestive mechanism goes into hibernation. If you slowly reintroduce food towards the conclusion of your fast, you will feel the healthiest.

- **Advantages**

Extended fasts, when appropriately overseen by a medical practitioner, may assist a person with obesity-related health problems. The longer fasting period maintains low sugar levels, which may be necessary for blood sugar issues to be overcome.

- **Disadvantages**

You will be famished for many days, which could cause problems with family meals and social occasions. Fasting for an extended period of time should be monitored, particularly when you are taking drugs that are influenced by your food. If you have diabetes and are fasting, your insulin will also need to be changed starting on the first day of the fast.

3.11. Meal Skipping

Meal skipping is an incredibly adaptable kind of IF that offers all the advantages of IF but with fewer restrictions. If you do not have a regular schedule or do not think a tighter version of the IF Diet would work for you, meal skipping is an option.

Meal skipping is a terrific approach for many individuals to respond to their bodies and follow their natural impulses. They just do not eat that meal if they are not hungry.

It is crucial to remember that when you miss meals, you will not always be fasting for the whole 10-16 hours. As a consequence, you may not get all of the benefits of other fasting diets. However, for individuals who desire a more natural intermittent fasting diet, this might be a good option. Perhaps it is a good idea for individuals who want to start paying more attention to their bodies so that they may transition to a more rigorous diet with ease. If you are not ready to plunge into one of these fasting diets just yet, it might be a terrific transitional diet for you

Chapter 4: How to Start Fasting and What to Expect?

It is your fifties. It is time to keep living a healthy lifestyle. As you go into the next phase of your life, your body requires to be adjusted in some manner. In this section, we will go over some basic changes that you should be aware of, such as various types of fasting as well as what fasting may do for you.

4.1. How it Works?

Fasting has been practiced by practically all faiths for centuries. Fasting has thus been practiced for almost 2,500 years. It is reasonable to think that if anything has been in use for this long, it must be having an impact on the lives of those who use it. Researchers from The National Weight Control Registry (NWCR) released a study in February 2007 that looked at 5,871 people who were devoted to their weight reduction program for 20 years and tracked their progress every three years. Researchers discovered that those who were willing to adopt this fasting lifestyle dropped an average of 13 pounds in only a few weeks. Their total weight and waist circumference both reduced by 2.3 cm. Fasting was shown to be helpful for both males and females, and their weight loss was not only safe but also successful.

4.2. States of Fasting

Depending on the length of time you fast, your body goes through many stages of the fed-fast cycle when you practice intermittent fasting.

4.2.1 The Fed state

After a meal, your body is in the absorptive stage, or fed state, when it is decomposing the food and collecting the nutrients. When you put the food in your mouth, it is torn down into its basic elements and absorbed into the gut, which is when digestion occurs.

4.2.2 The early fasting state

Several hours after eating, blood glucose levels drop, resulting in a reduction in insulin production and an increase in glucagon production; glucagon is released by pancreatic cells in order to respond to low blood sugar in the fasting phase.

4.2.3 The fasting state

After food has been digested, processed, and stored, the post-absorptive state, often known as the fasting state, occurs. Fasting overnight is typical, but missing meals throughout the day also keep your body in this condition. The body must depend on stored glycogen to keep going in this situation.

4.2.4 Long-term fasting state (Starvation state)

Adipose tissue begins to lose mass if more energy is spent than is absorbed. Both insulin and leptin secretion decrease under these circumstances, fuel utilization rises, and energy reserves are depleted. When calories are ingested in excess, the opposite is true.

4.3. Why it is Effective?

Fasting works so successfully for so many individuals because it restores the internal clock, which is really the timekeeper for almost all your body's operations, including digestion, insulin regulation, and so on. Fasting adjusts the internal clock in such a manner that it helps the body to burn fat more efficiently, reducing fat accumulation and the risk of diabetes. It is crucial to remember, too, that fasting is not really something you should do every day. It is really advised that you are doing it once a month or once a season. Although there are certain advantages to doing this regularly, for at least one month, you should stick to the guideline of just doing it once a month.

4.4. How to do it?

If you go to fast once a month for roughly 24 hours, begin with a 12-h fast. This implies you will only eat in the 12 hours leading up to your regular lunchtime. You should also avoid eating after 18:00. This implies that if your supper time is 22:00, you should not consume anything after 18:00. By following these guidelines, you will be ready to get all the advantages of fasting while avoiding any bad consequences. It is critical for individuals who are just getting started with this sort of dieting approach to take a sit back and realize what they are doing since anything more than 24 hours may be unsafe and lead to major health issues.

4.5. Changing Your Diet

It is critical to alter your meals in order to maximize the benefits of fasting. The body's ability to burn fat decreases as you grow older. This implies that adjusting your food rather than relying on your body to adjust is a far better approach. Elimination of simple carbs and sugars is one of the first things you will want to think about. These meals will cause your blood sugar to rise, making it harder for your body to keep them stable. You should also consume as much fiber as possible. Fiber is beneficial to your digestive system and has a significant impact. It is also crucial to drink enough liquid - at least 1.5 liters every day - in addition to modifying your eating habits (more if possible). Water will help you stay hydrated while also flushing pollutants out of your system. It is also crucial to get adequate salt intake as part of this. Adults should consume around 2 grams of salt each day (more if feasible), but keep in mind that you will require more salt while fasting than usual since your body cannot retain water without salt. It is also vital to limit your salt intake in addition to avoiding simple sweets and carbs. You should also be able to acquire sufficient potassium in your meals under typical conditions (as long as you consume enough veggies). However, to have any impact on your body when fasting, you will need some more salt than usual. This implies you should add extra potassium to your meal rather than salt. Skin-on potatoes, bananas, tomatoes, raisins, leafy greens, and broccoli are all good sources of potassium.

4.6. Prepare Your Body to Feel Different

On days 2 and 3 of any fast, many individuals feel exhausted, have a headache, and are generally "out of sorts." That is quite typical. Fasting's unpleasant side effects usually fade away by the third or fourth day. If you are fasting for less than two days, you will probably find relief as soon as the fast is through. After the unpleasant effects have subsided on day three, most individuals feel terrific, with a feeling of calmness, well-being, and heightened attention taking over. However, if you sense anything is wrong with you during your fast, other than being tired, you should absolutely eat. You can always give it another shot.

Chapter 5: How to Track Progress While Fasting?

Counting down the hours before you can bite into another sandwich—or keeping a record of your 500 calories on each of your fasting days—may be a bit of a grind if you are just getting started with IF, regardless matter which strategy you choose. Of course, there are apps for that. Among the most prominent intermittent fasting applications are:

- Zero®

- FastHabit Intermittent Fasting®

- LIFE Fasting Tracker®

- Window®

- YouAte Food & Health Diary®

- BodyFast®

- Vora®

- Fastient®

- Simple®

- Femometer Fasting®

5.1. Zero®

Cost: Free

Zero is a simple tracker that lets you pick a daily fasting technique like 16:8 or a fasting duration of up to 24 hours. There is a clock that ticks down or up (depending on your preference) and keeps track of how many hours you have fasted for the preceding seven days. This program is basic and straightforward to use.

It is a good monitoring software if your fasting routine is consistent every day, and it can help you commit to regular intermittent fasting. If your usual fasting time varies from day to day, then it is not recommended. It delivers alerts to your smartphone or Smartwatch regarding your fasting beginning and end timings, which is a useful tool for keeping you responsible.

5.2. FastHabit Intermittent Fasting®

Cost: Free

The FastHabit application is ideal for every kind of fasting, whether you fast for the same amount of hours every day or whether your fasting window varies. It works, for example, if you follow the 16:8 or 5:2 diet and wish to have a reduced eating period on those two days.

It enables you to choose the duration of your fasting timeframe, which you may change once it has started. You may also include a fast from the previous day. There is a timer that counts the hours until your fast finishes, so glancing at it might motivate you to keep going even if you just have a few hours left.

You can also view an overview of the previous ten days, which may help urge you to keep to your daily fasting plan and set reminders for when a fast begins or finishes, which will send alerts to your mobile or Smartwatch.

5.3. LIFE Fasting Tracker®

Cost: Free

Since you can specify the start and finish times as well as objectives for how long you like to fast, the LIFE IF software enables you to monitor your success on any fasting plan. A clock displays the minutes and hours fasted, and a short peek might make you feel pleased with how long you have fasted.

This application also tracks the total time you have fasted and how many fasts you have had, as well as your weekly fasting statistics. If you have fasting partners who also use this app, you may fast simultaneously, and the encouragement may help you adhere to your diet.

5.4. Window®

Cost: $2.99

Window is a weight-loss tool that lets you manage your regular fasting window and measure your success over time. You may also check a monthly calendar summary that displays how often you have fasted per day, which might motivate you to keep up with your regular fasting routine.

5.5. YouAte Food and Health Diary®

Cost: Free

YouAte is a visual meal notebook that lets you capture images of what you ate when, how you felt while eating it, and how much time has passed between snacks and meals. This might help you realize why you overeat or choose bad food during your meal window and motivate healthier eating habits

5.6. BodyFast®

Cost: Free

BodyFast is an online IF platform established in Germany. It is one of the top fasting apps because of its unique and diverse fasting strategies. Users may choose a trainer and follow his balanced diet advice. To remain competitive and motivated, the user may upgrade and participate in weekly challenges.

The application has a FAQs section that covers the majority of the frequently asked issues regarding IF for beginners. To date, nearly 8 million individuals use the fasting tracker on a regular basis

5.7. Vora®

Cost: Free

This software tracks daily fasting/goal times as well as weight reduction. If you are seeking a weight reduction app with comparable functionality, Vora is a good option. Vora is the finest intermittent fasting software since it is cloud-based and enables users to create, update, and cancel fasts.

Users may see their last seven fasts in a stunning chart that illustrates their progress toward their goals. The Vora app enables users to choose their own fasting pattern, ranging from a complete fast to a 5:2 or alternate day diet. So far, the application has amassed a community of approximately 3, 00,000 fasters

5.8. Fastient®

Cost: Free

A meal schedule and food intake records are required to maintain discipline during fasting. The Fastient app provides a large, open layout with lots of areas for a user's diary; users can examine data in simple graphs and quickly enter their food intake using the fasting timetable tracker.

5.9. Simple®

Cost: $15 per month

Simple is an app that does exactly what it says: it simplifies intermittent fasting. Moreover, this software will assist you in managing your fasting intervals and reminding you when it is time to eat, mentoring you throughout the day with notifications and some old-fashioned smartphone inspiration through frequent fasting suggestions. Simple will notify you what to do when, as well as giving push alerts for water intake to keep you on target with your hydration. This software will react to your behavior over time using a fast adaptive tracker, allowing you to keep to your fasting regimen and new habits.

You may register for a free Simple account or pay for a premium account. Both Apple and Android smartphones are supported by the app.

5.10. Femometer Fasting®

Cost: Free for a basic account

Femometer Fasting is an amazing app for anybody who enjoys studying the details of what happens on an IF diet. Femometer Fasting is a simple app that tracks your fasting durations and reminds you when it is time to eat. The application also motivates you to track your fasting hours as well as other lifestyle factors such as sleep schedule, exercise activity and food and water consumption. All these information points add up to a "Body Status," which gives you insight into what is going on within your body when you are fasting. You may find out when you will start burning fat for fuel, receive nutritional instruction, and more.

Femometer Fasting is accessible with a free account, but for $9.99 per month, $14.99 for three months, or $49.99 yearly, you may switch to a premium membership. The software is currently only accessible on Apple's iOS platform.

Chapter 6: Safety and Side Effects of Intermittent Fasting

If you are thinking about experiencing intermittent fasting, you are undoubtedly wondering if it has any negative consequences. For most women over 50, modified variations of intermittent fasting seem to be safe.

6.1 How Safe is Intermittent Fasting for Women?

If done correctly, IF for women may be extremely helpful. If calories are controlled too severely, it might cause hormonal imbalances, which may lead to irregular periods and infertility.

Women who choose IF should pay attention to their diet's nutritional quality. Otherwise, individuals risk losing the advantages of IF and doing more damage to their bodies than good.

Note: Before attempting intermittent fasting, ask your doctor if you have a medical issue.

Medical advice is especially necessary for women who:

- Have had an eating disorder in the past.

- Have diabetes or suffer from low blood sugar on a regular basis.

- Are underweight, malnourished, or deficient in nutrients.

- Suffer from infertility or have a record of amenorrhea (missed periods).

Finally, intermittent fasting seems to have a favorable safety profile. However, if you have any issues, such as a lack of your menstrual period, you should stop immediately.

6.2 Side Effects

Intermittent fasting has been found in studies to have some mild adverse effects and is not the best option for everyone.

6.2.1. Hunger and cravings

Hunger is probably one of the main prevalent negative effects of intermittent fasting. You may feel greater hunger if you limit your food intake or go for long periods without eating.

Some of the 112 adults who took part in the trial were allocated to an intermittent energy restriction team. For a year, they ingested 400 to 600 calories on two non-consecutive days each week. These people had greater hunger levels than individuals who ate a low-calorie diet and restricted their calories on a regular basis.

According to studies, hunger is a condition that most individuals feel during the first few days of a fasting program. A 2020 research looked at 1,422 participants who fasted for 4–21 days. They only had hunger sensations over the first several days of the routines. As your body adjusts to regular fasting periods, sensations like hunger may fade.

6.2.2. Digestive issues

If you undertake intermittent fasting, you may encounter digestive disorders such as constipation, diarrhea, nausea, and bloating. The decrease in food intake that various intermittent fasting regimes entail may have a severe impact on your digestion, resulting in constipation and other unpleasant side effects. Additionally, dietary modifications connected with intermittent fasting regimens might result in bloating and diarrhea.

Constipation may be exacerbated by dehydration, another typical adverse effect of intermittent fasting. As a result, it is critical to keep properly hydrated when fasting intermittently. Constipation may be avoided by eating nutrient-dense, high-fiber meals.

6.2.3. Dehydration

As previously stated, the body discharges a huge amount of water as well as salt in the urine during the first few days of fasting. Natural diuresis, also known as fasting natriuresis, is the name given to this process. You might get dehydrated if this occurs to you and you do not restore the water and electrolytes you lost via urination.

In addition, those who practice IF may neglect to drink or drink insufficiently. This is particularly true when you initially start an intermittent fasting program.

Drink fluids during the day and keep an eye on the color of your urine to remain adequately hydrated. It should ideally be the hue of light lemonade. You may be dehydrated if your urine is black in color.

6.2.4. Headaches and lightheadedness

Intermittent fasting is often associated with headaches. They usually happen in the initial few days of a fasting regimen.

In a study published in 2020, researchers looked at 18 papers, including persons who practiced intermittent fasting. Some individuals in the four trials who reported adverse effects indicated they experienced minor headaches.

Researchers have discovered that "fasting headaches" are frequently situated in the frontal area of the brain, with pain that is mild to moderate in severity.

Furthermore, persons who suffer from headaches often are more likely to suffer from headaches when fasting than those who do not. Lower blood sugar and caffeine withdrawal, according to research, may lead to headaches during IF.

6.2.5. Fatigue and low energy

Some individuals who practice different forms of intermittent fasting report weariness and poor energy levels, according to studies. Intermittent fasting might make you feel fatigued and weak due to low blood sugar. In addition, intermittent fasting may produce sleep disruptions in certain persons, resulting in fatigue throughout the day.

Intermittent fasting, on the other hand, has been shown in some studies to decrease tiredness, particularly when your body adapts to regular fasting intervals.

6.2.6. Sleep disturbances

According to some studies, insomnia, such as the inability to fall or remain asleep, are one of the most prevalent negative effects of intermittent fasting.

In a 2020 research, 1,422 participants took part in fasting regimes that lasted 4–21 days. Fasting caused sleep disruptions in 15% of the subjects, according to the research. This was mentioned more often than other negative effects.

Because your body excretes huge quantities of salt and water via the urine, fatigue is more typical in the early days of an IF diet. Dehydration and low salt levels might occur as a result of this.

Other experiments, on the other hand, have found that intermittent fasting has no impact on sleep. Research published in 2021 looked at 31 obese persons who fasted on alternate days while simultaneously eating a low-carb diet for six months. The research discovered that this regimen had no effect on sleep quality, duration, or the severity of insomnia.

6.2.7. Malnutrition

Intermittent fasting, if done incorrectly, may result in malnutrition. Malnutrition may occur when a person fasts for lengthy periods of time and does not refill their body with necessary nutrients. The same may be said for unplanned, long-term energy restriction diets.

On different forms of intermittent fasting regimens, people are often able to satisfy their calorie and nutritional demands. However, if you do not properly plan or follow your fasting program over a lengthy length of time, or if you purposely limit calories to an excessive degree, you risk malnutrition and other health problems. That is why, while fasting intermittently, it is critical to eat a well-balanced, healthy diet. Make sure you are not restricting your calorie intake too much.

A healthcare expert who is familiar with intermittent fasting can assist you in developing a safe diet that offers the optimum quantity of calories and nutrients for you.

6.2.8. Bad breath

During intermittent fasting, some individuals may have bad breath as a side effect. A deficiency of salivary circulation and an increase in acetone in the breath cause this.

When you fast, your body burns fat as a source of energy. Because acetone is a byproduct of fat metabolism, it accumulates in the blood and breath while you fast. Dehydration may result in a dry mouth, which can produce bad breath.

6.2.9. Irritability and other mood changes

When individuals practice intermittent fasting, they may suffer irritation and other mood swings. If your blood sugar levels are low, you may get irritable.

Hypoglycemia, or low blood sugar, may occur during times of dietary changes or fasting. Irritability, anxiousness, and poor focus are all possible outcomes. Fasting raises cortisol levels in women, according to research. In addition to becoming more stressed, hunger caused by fasting may make women irritable and unhappy.

Interestingly, the researchers discovered that, though the ladies were irritated towards the conclusion of the fasting period, they also felt a greater feeling of accomplishment, pride, and self-control than they did at the beginning.

6.2.10. Risk of Hypoglycemia

Low blood sugar is known as hypoglycemia, and it becomes more likely the more you go without eating. While our systems are designed to fast overnight, they are not necessarily designed to go without food for more than 8-10 hours. Fasting also increases the possibility of low blood sugar if you previously have a problem with it.

Regardless of the causes or side effects that women over 50 suffer when they begin fasting, it is a fantastic remedial approach since it helps to prevent or decrease virtually all of the age-related illnesses that women over 50 suffer. It also aids in maintaining healthy body weight.

Chapter 7: The Role of Exercise and Active Lifestyle in Weight Loss

It is fantastic if you were healthy and active before the age of 50. But it is not too late to begin exercising consistently if you have not already.

Hot flashes, joint discomfort, and sleep issues are some of the indicators of menopause that may be alleviated via physical exercise. Exercise may also help prevent heart problems, diabetes, and osteoporosis. It also aids weight loss and burns abdominal fat. Exercise has such powerful benefits that it improves every physiological system of the body.

7.1. Staying Fit as You Age

Many aging problems are connected to a sedentary lifestyle. While your actual age maybe fifty-five, your biological age might be thirty-five if you stick to a regular workout routine. Consult your doctor before beginning, particularly if you have any of the heart disease risk factors. Then it is time to begin going.

- **Physical health benefits of exercise for seniors**

Exercise may help you maintain or decrease weight as an adult woman.

- Maintain or lose weightz

Managing a healthy weight might be difficult when your metabolism slows as you get older. Regular exercise helps your body burn more calories by increasing your metabolism and building muscle mass.

- Reduce the impact of illness and chronic disease

Greatly reduce the negative effects of sickness and chronic disease. Exercise improves immunological and digestive function, BP and bone density and reduces the risk of Alzheimer's illness, diabetes, overweight, cardiovascular disease, osteoporosis, and some malignancies in people.

- Enhance your mobility, flexibility, and balance

Improve your flexibility, mobility, and balance. Exercise increases your stamina, agility, and posture, which may assist with balance and coordination while also lowering your chance of falling. Strength training may also assist with the symptoms of long-term illnesses like arthritis.

- **Mental health benefits of exercise**

Exercise may also help you:

- Get a better night's sleep

As you become older, getting enough sleep becomes more

important for your general health. Regular exercise may assist you in falling asleep more quickly, sleeping more deeply, and waking up feeling more energized and refreshed.

o **Improve your mood and self-confidence**

Exercise is a fantastic stress reliever, and the endorphins released may really assist in alleviating melancholy, tension, and anxiety. Being active and powerful might also make you feel more self-assured.

o **Enhance your cognitive abilities**

Sudoku and crossword puzzles are good ways to keep your brain engaged, but nothing compares to the benefits of exercise on the brain. It may assist with multitasking and creativity in the brain, as well as memory problems, cognitive loss, and dementia. Staying active may even assist in halting the development of brain diseases like Alzheimer's.

7.2. Types of Exercises

Not all workouts are affected equally, so make sure your training program includes a variety of them. The following are the four major types of exercise:

• **Strengthening exercises**

Lifting weights and resistance-based exercises, like Pilates or resistance band workouts, are good weight-training programs for women over 50.

- **Aerobic/cardiovascular exercise**

Aerobic or cardiovascular activities are sometimes known as endurance exercises since they must be done for at least 10 minutes. While you are breathing and your heart rate should rise during aerobic activity, you may still be able to communicate with a workout partner. Aerobic exercise includes things like walking, running, and swimming.

- **Stretching**

Stretching exercises assist in increasing or maintain flexibility, which reduces the chance of muscle or joint damage. Yoga is a well-known stretching activity.

- **Balance**

The danger of falling rises as you become older. Falls may be reduced by doing exercises that help you improve or maintain your balance. Balancing on one foot may be an easy balancing exercise.

Even though there are four different types of exercise, it is vital to remember that workout does not exist in a vacuum. When you walk, for example, you are not just increasing your cardiovascular system but also developing your leg muscles.

Some strength training routines may also be used to stretch muscles and enhance balance.

7.3. Exercises Suitable for Women Over 50

Among the most prominent exercises suitable for women over 50 are:

- Knee push-ups

- Basic squat

- Forward lunge with Bicep curl

- Shoulder overhead press

- Reverse Grip Double Arm Row

- Plank Pose

- Chest Fly

- Single-Leg Hamstring Bridge

- Stability Ball Side Leg Lift

- Basic Ab

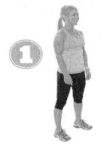
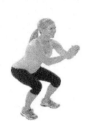

BASIC SQUATS

KNEE PUSH-UPS

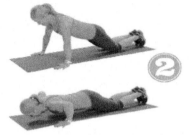

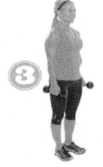
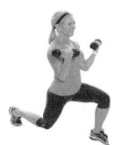

FORWARD LUNGE WITH BICEP CURL

SHOULDER OVERHEAD PRESS

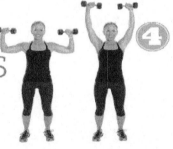

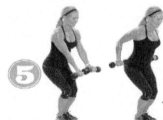

REVERSE GRIP DOUBLE ARM ROW

7.3.1. Knee push-ups

Instructions

- Begin in a kneeling posture with both hands on the floor, slightly wider than the breadth of your shoulders. Keep your knees behind your hips at all times.

- Maintain a long neck and use your glutes and inner thighs to keep your lower body engaged.

- Slowly lower yourself to the ground, bringing your chest near it. Maintain a 45-degree angle with your elbows while you perform this.

- Return to the beginning posture by pushing yourself up.

- A rep for a total of 20 times, or as many as you feel comfortable with.

You may attempt the full push-up variation after you have mastered the knee push-ups. For the complete version, your toes will be the only ones touching the floor instead of your knees. Then, do it as many times as you can and gradually improve your performance.

7.3.2. Basic Squat

Instructions

- Begin by kneeling with your hands underneath your shoulders and your knees behind your hips.

- Maintain a long neck by maintaining your eyes next to your fingers and press your inner thighs and glutes together to keep your lower body active.

- Slowly drop yourself to the floor, maintaining a 45-degree angle with your elbows.

- Return to the beginning posture by pushing yourself up.

- Repeat for the appropriate number of times.

7.3.3. Forward lunge with bicep curl

Instructions

- Maintain a tall posture and your feet hip-distance apart. With one foot, take a big stride forward and drop your body to the ground. At the bottom of the lunge, both legs must be bent at a 90-degree.

- To complete a bicep curl, bring the weights in towards the shoulders, then push off the front foot and come back to the beginning.

- Switch sides and repeat the process.

7.3.4. Knee push-ups

Instructions

- Maintain a straight back and stand tall.

- With an overhand grip, grab a dumbbell in both hands at the shoulders. Knuckles should be facing up, and thumbs must be on the inside.

- Exhale as you raise the weights over your head in a steady manner at the apex of the motion, pause.

- While inhaling, return the weights to the shoulders.

- As desired, perform for eight to twelve repetitions.

7.3.5. Reverse grip double arm row

Instructions

- Begin by sitting back into a small squat with your legs together, working your glutes and abdomen. Arms will be extended out to the body, palms toward the ceiling, grasping the weights.

- By pressing the upper back muscles collectively, draw your elbows back and slowly lift them beyond your hips until you sense the triceps and lats engaged. Return to the beginning position with control.

Option: Begin with lesser weights and concentrate on steady, controlled motions. At the apex of the range of motion, take a 3-second pause before gently returning to the initial position. Grab a set of larger weights and attempt completing a few extra reps after you have mastered lesser weights with a moderate and controlled pace.

7.3.6. Plank pose

Instructions

The plank may help you not only build and tone your core muscles (abdominal and lower back muscles), but it may also help you enhance your balance. Planks may also help you

improve your stance, which is beneficial if you spend most of your day sitting on a desk chair. There are a few different methods to do a plank.

- To do a **high plank**, go into a posture where your legs and arms are straight as if you were at the peak of a push-up.

- A **low plank** is another alternative, which is simpler to accomplish if you are a novice. Instead of leaning on the hands, bend both arms at the elbows and lean on your forearms to support your weight.

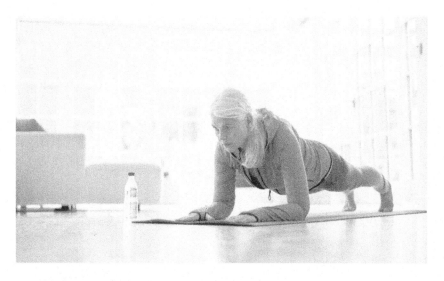

Note: Keep your back totally straight as your head up no matter which option you pick. Make a straight line with your whole-body parallel to the floor.

7.3.7. Chest fly

Instructions

- The chest muscles of women are often weak and undeveloped. The chest fly is a powerlifting exercise that helps those muscles get stronger.

- A set of hand weights is required for this workout. Lie flat on your back, knees bent, feet planted on the floor. Lift both arms over your chest, holding one dumbbell in each hand.

- Slowly open your arms to the sides, dropping the arms and wrists to the floor but without touching them. So that your arms do not lockout, keep your elbows bent slightly. Repeat by raising your arms again.

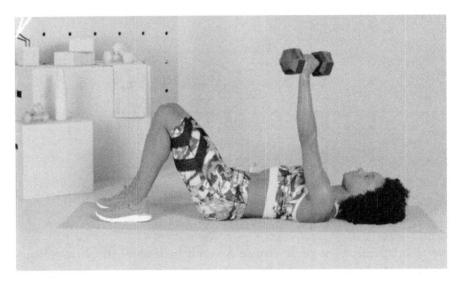

7.3.8. Single leg hamstring bridge

Instructions

- Lie down on your back with your knees bent and your feet flat on the ground, with your knees, hip-distance apart.

- Raise hips off the surface into a bridge by squeezing glutes. For 8-12 repetitions, lower and elevate the hips, then switch sides.

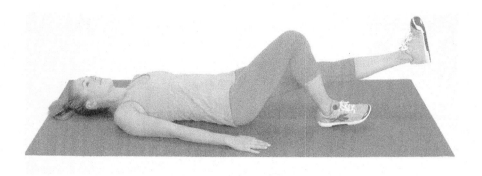

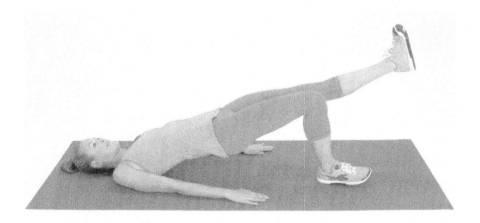

7.3.9. Stability ball side leg lift

Instructions

- Kneel on your right side with the ball.

- Allow your right side to lean on the ball and embrace it with your right arm.

- Extend the left leg to the side as far as it will go. On the floor, keep the right leg bent.

- 8 – 12 times, slowly raise and drop your left leg, then swap sides.

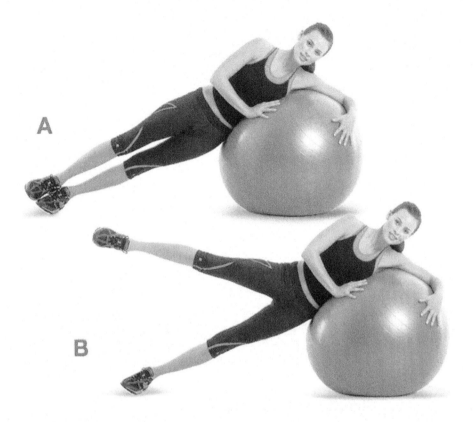

7.3.10. Basic Ab

Instructions

"Women over 50 are more likely to acquire a bloated belly," Perkins adds. "This technique is excellent for drawing your abdominal muscles inside into your spine, strengthening and tightening them."

- Lie down on your back, feet on the floor, knees bent at a 90-degree at the back of the knees.

- Keeping your upper body relaxed, position both hands on your thighs. Gradually lower your chin towards the chest and raise your shoulders off the floor as you exhale.

- Your hands will rise near your knees as you do so. Continue to raise your shoulders until your fingers reach your knees or your shoulders are totally off the floor.

- Pause for 2 seconds at the peak, then gently fall back to the initial position. That is the first time you have done it. Aim for a total of 20 to 30 repetitions.

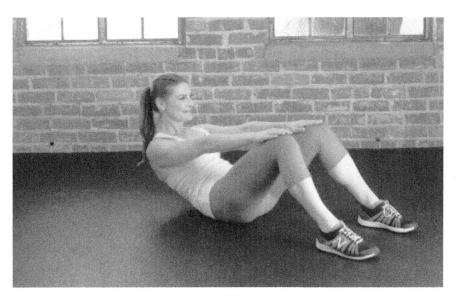

Chapter 8: Life-Changing Proven Tips and Tricks to Stay Healthy and Common Mistakes to Avoid

A solid offense is the best defense. Long-term health is the outcome of a good defense — proactive, preventive, and healthy choices that affect your health presently, tomorrow, and in the future. Start early if you want to mature gracefully. Start with being a healthy, vibrant younger person if you wish to be a healthy, active older person.

Good health is not a fluke; it is the consequence of a lifetime of good practices. You may guarantee that you not only survive long but also live well by developing healthy habits today. Start by modifying the small decisions you make every day to guarantee your physical and mental wellness as you age.

8.1. Tricks and Tips for Staying Healthy After 50

The more you grow older, the more you realize how important it is to look for oneself. That involves quitting smoking, eating well, and exercising regularly. Improving your mouth's health is critical for avoiding a variety of issues, including diabetes and heart disease. It is not too late to priorities your health. Here are a few things to consider if you are over 50:

- **Drink plenty of water**

When you are fasting, water keeps the body hydrated and helps you feel fuller. Fasting also has the effect of acting as a diuretic, which means your body will typically remove fluids at a higher pace than usual. What it comes down to is that for the optimum effects, you should strive to drink a gallon of fresh water every day. Tea and coffee should be consumed: When you are hungry, you may discover that drinking tea or coffee helps to suppress your appetite. Caffeine is an appetite suppressor that is found in nature. Caffeine should not be used too close to sleep, or you may experience difficulties sleeping.

- **Keep yourself busy**

You will discover that you are more productive while you are hungry. You will not only get more done if you keep yourself occupied, but you will also be able to divert yourself from the cravings. If you do not find constructive methods to pass the time, particularly initially, the hours you are fasting will appear to extend out into days. Do not make things any more difficult for yourself than they have to be. Ensure your days are jam-packed with activities in the early stages of your changed eating habit.

- **Make it flexible**

Intermittent fasting provides a plethora of benefits. You are not obligated to choose one choice simply because everyone else does. You may mix and combine to come up with a timetable that suits your needs. It is more about having the flexibility to do it your way when it comes to intermittent fasting.

- **Try it for at least a month**

To see whether the IF is suitable for you, you will need to try it for at least four weeks. If you are not doing it for this long, your body will not be able to adjust, and you will not be giving it a full chance to see whether it is the best decision for you; give it at least this length of time to try it out.

- **Experiment with fasting methods**

It is possible that what works on one individual will not work for you. If you discover that specific fasting hours or a certain kind of intermittent fasting works better for you, go with that. It is all about experimenting to find out what works best for you.

- **Delay your breakfast slowly**

Many individuals find that gradually delaying breakfast works well for them. By progressively moving your breakfast time back to 1 hour each week or so, you will be able to transition to an IF without too much difficulty. For example, if you normally have breakfast at 8 a.m., you should wait until 8:30 a.m. during the first week. Then, in week 2, move your breakfast up to 9 a.m. Carry on like this until your first meal, which should be about midday.

- **Drink water in the morning**

The fact that you went the entire night without eating is often the cause of your morning hunger. Drinking one glass of water first thing in the morning is a wonderful habit to get into.

- **Add weights**

If you want to reduce weight or tone up, adding weight exercise to your program makes sense. While you should not change things up too frequently when you are first starting out, after your body has adjusted to an IF lifestyle, there is no reason why you should not. You will be shocked at what your body is capable of. If you start cautiously, you should ultimately be able to endure a full-intensity exercise without being too exhausted to function afterward.

- **Live it up**

When it comes to intermittent fasting, you must know that you may overeat on occasion. You may have a good time if everything levels out in the end. While most diets focus on the items you are not permitted to consume; intermittent fasting takes into consideration the reality that you cannot always plan your meals. This implies that if you get your fasting time in, there is no reason you should not be able to shift your hours about sometimes. Furthermore, there is no reason why you should not treat yourself every now and again if one indulgent dessert does not grow into seven or eight.

- **Get out of the house**

In your house, there is plenty of temptation. As a result, it is preferable to go out of the home so that you do not eat most of that food. Even if you have children, come up with an activity that you can all do to keep yourself engaged.

- **Eat more protein and healthy fat**

It is simpler to manage your hunger and grow muscle mass if you eat more protein with each meal. The healthier fat in your diet will give you more energy and make you feel satiated for longer. The gradual growth of the Typical American Diet has resulted in the great majority of people in western Countries eating far too many carbs and much too little protein or good fat. Start thinking about the macros of the meals you consume to solve this issue. Also, pack your plate with things that will make stretching it out to the upcoming window as simple as possible while you are in an eating window.

- **Avoid the bad stuff**

Make sure you are not using this as a reason to consume junk food all the time. Even if you want to fast, make sure you stick to a well-balanced diet to ensure your body gets adequate nourishment. It is crucial to remember that a key aspect of IF is creating a calorie deficit at the ending of the week to help you lose even more weight. As a result, when you enter an eating window and stuff your body with high-calorie junk food, you are essentially ruining all your personal effort. Making healthy choices all the time will ensure that your weight reduction efforts are more successful overall.

As you have seen, there are a variety of ways to maximize the benefits of intermittent fasting. However, no matter how severe your fasting is, you should not expect to lose weight on a consistent basis. While you will most likely lose weight initially as your body adjusts to having fewer calories in its system, this will likely come and go during your fasting period. The consequences are most evident during the early few weeks of the shift, as your body attempts to hang on to whatever it has until it can sort out what is going on. Things should, however, progress as planned once it gets into the swing of things.

Every diet will have weight reduction plateaus at some point. That is just an unavoidable aspect of losing weight. Weight reduction will ultimately resume if you remain steady. Trying to switch things up to get your weight reduction back on track is the worst option you can do since it will just make it more challenging for your body to lose weight again. Instead, if you stick with it and do your best, you will start noticing improvements again before you realize it.

8.2. Common Mistakes to Avoid During Intermittent Fasting

Intermittent fasting has different effects on different people, but in general, everyone should be able to benefit from it in some way. The goal is to execute it correctly and consistently. Here are some frequent blunders that might jeopardize your results:

- **Starting with an Extreme Plan**

Don't you want to dive in with all your excitement and kick the hell out of it now that you have discovered a fasting strategy that seems just right for your needs? You are probably already envisioning your new appearance after you have lost the weight. Is it possible to begin fasting right now? No. Allowing your enthusiasm to mislead you to an extreme strategy that will drastically alter your physique is not a good idea. You cannot go from three meals a day plus snacks to a 24-hour fast. You will be unhappy as a result of this. Begin by skipping individual meals. Alternatively, avoiding snacking. Once your body has become used to brief fasts, you may go as far as your health will allow, within reason. Exercise slowly during the fasting period, at least in the first several weeks since it may promote Adrenal Fatigue.

• **Quitting Too Soon**

So, you have been fasting for one week and already thought it is too difficult? Do you have hunger pains, cravings, mood swings, poor energy, and other issues? Such a response is to be expected, after all. As the body adapts to the lower calorie intake, the first few weeks might be difficult. You will feel hungry, angry, and tired. You must, however, maintain your consistency. The body is adjusting to the changes, even if you cannot feel them. If you quit during this time and go back to your old eating habits, you will undo the changes your body has already made. Any change, even this one, needs discipline. Hold on; things will improve with time.

• **Feasting Too Much**

Intermittent fasting is stated as a period of fasting followed by a period of feasting by some quarters. This essentially means that as soon as the bell rings the very last moment of fast time, you dive into a massive savory meal, the type that ends with a loud, satisfying belch. After all, you have managed it through your fasting window, so there should not be anything wrong with this strategy.

But keep in mind that the primary objective here is to reduce weight and burn fat. This is only effective if you consume fewer calories than you expend. The greater the size of your meal, the more calories you are putting into your body. You do not have to consume a mountain of food. Beginning with vegetables and fruits is a good place to start. They include fiber, which makes you feel filled, so you will not have to eat as much. Slowly eat, paying attention to the signs that you are full. Finish dining as soon as you are satisfied, even if there is still stuff on your plate from the hunger you have been experiencing. Keep the leftovers in the fridge for another supper. You also do not have to eat until the end of the eating window. Go on and focus on other things after you are pleased.

- **Insufficient Calories**

While some people would overeat to try and compensate for the 'time lost,' others will eat so little to avoid undoing their gains. This results in insufficient Calories, even though these Calories are essential to power the body's functioning at its best. You are more prone to suffer mood fluctuations, irritation, weariness, and poor energy levels if you do not get enough nutrition. Your daily life will be disrupted, and you will be less active as a result; fasting should improve your life, not make it worse. You will be able to stay active and complete your fasting plan more quickly if you eat enough.

- **Wrong Food Choices**

We have previously learned that intermittent fasting focuses on the when rather than what when it comes to eating. While this still allows you to sample a broad range of meals, it does not imply that you are free to eat everything you want. If we are allowed to our own ways, most of us will choose sweet and fatty meals because they appeal to our taste senses. Sandwich, dessert, pastries, chocolates, ice cream, and processed meats are just a few examples. However, this is a rather short-sighted attitude. Ending your fast with these meals will simply negate the fast's advantages.

Choose healthful, whole meals that will provide the body with all the nutrients it needs. Vegetables, protein, healthy fats, and complex carbohydrates should all be included in your meal. You may have noticed that IF and a low-carb diet go well together. Yes, but this is a limited-carb, not a no-carb. Some individuals attempt to lose weight faster by cutting off all carbohydrates. Carbs provide you with calories to power your body. On your plate, include a piece of nutritious starch, preferably unprocessed brown choices. Why should you be concerned with what you eat when intermittent fasting is concerned with when you eat? Healthy nutrition is important for everybody, even if you are not on a fasting regimen. You consume healthy meals since they are excellent for your body and protect you from developing lifestyle disorders. Regular eating should be healthy eating; thus, we may conclude that fast is complemented with normal eating in this scenario.

- **Insufficient Fluids**

It is easier to stick to your fast if you stay hydrated. It gives you a sensation of fullness and keeps hunger at bay. Fasting also helps the body break down damaged components, and the liquid aids filter these out as toxins. You may also drink tea or coffee without adding milk or sugar. Coffee has been shown to have chemicals that help the body burn fat faster. Green tea has comparable qualities to black tea. You may experiment with different tea or coffee tastes to find one that you like. They are fine as long as they do not contain any calories.

- **Over-Concentrating on the Eating Window**

You are not handling it correctly unless you cannot keep your gaze away from the clock. You cannot pass the fasting period daydreaming about food, planning how much and what you will eat when the time comes. The more you worry about eating, the hungrier you get. Emotional hunger is the hunger you experience after 5 hours or so. It is clock hunger, and you will notice it around mealtimes. If you have been fasting for at least 16 hours, true hunger sets in. Take your thoughts away from eating and focus on anything else. If you are at home and find yourself circling the kitchen, get out of there. Go to the museum, go shopping (but not for food), go to the park, or do errands. It is a lot simpler to stay away from food if it is out of sight.

- **Wrong Plan**

We have previously gone through the several fasting regimens that are available and the things to consider while picking one. This should help you fast in a relaxed manner. How do you realize your current strategy is not the greatest for you? The whole procedure becomes a tremendous burden, to begin with. Hunger, fatigue, mood fluctuations, and a lack of energy are all problems you face. Your work performance suffers, and you look forward to the next fast. And, despite all of the effort, there is nothing to speak for it. Return to the plans and select the one that best fits your needs.

- **Stress**

If you are experiencing a lot of stress, you will probably find it difficult to stick to the fast. Stress produces hormonal imbalances, causing hunger pains while you could have been fasting without difficulty. Stress eating is prevalent, and it is characterized by desires for fatty and sugary meals. It also disrupts sleep, making fasting even more difficult if you are not well-rested. If you had tried the fast before and made any of these errors, as many people do, you may fix yourself and continue. If you are just getting started, you now know what to avoid.

The goal is to keep growing and learning, and the outcomes will speak for themselves.

- **Managing Stress**

Because anxiety is one of the things that might affect your fasting, it is critical that you know how to cope with it.

Here are some actions you may take to guarantee that anxiety does not get in the way of enjoying a healthy lifestyle:

o **Relax Daily**

In the long term, the difficulties that you hold in your mind and heart might lead you to become anxious. So that the strain does not build up, find a method to relax at the end of each day. Watch a movie, a sporting event, a biography, read a book, attempt a new dish, take a bath, or do anything else that interests you. Those few hours give a welcome diversion, allowing you to focus on the issues of the day ahead without being distracted by those of the day before.

- **Go Easy on Yourself**

Accept that regardless of how hard you strive, you will never be able to achieve perfection. You also do not have complete control over your life. So, do yourself a favor and avoid overestimating your abilities. Also, remember to preserve your sense of humor. Humor helps a lot toward calming you down.

- **Talk About Your Problems**

If something is upsetting you, talking about it might help you relax. Relatives, friends, a trustworthy cleric, a doctor, or a psychologist are all good places to start. You may also converse with yourself. It is known as self-talk, and we all engage in it. However, in order for self-talk to be beneficial in reducing stress, it must be positive rather than negative.

So, when you are anxious, pay attention to what you are thinking or saying. Change the negative message you are sending yourself to a pleasant one. Do not tell yourself, "I can't do this," for example. Instead, tell yourself, "I can do this," or "I'm doing the most I can."

If you are having trouble figuring out what is causing your stress, consider maintaining a stress diary. Make a record of when you feel the most worried and discover if you can see a trend, then figure out how to eliminate or mitigate those triggers.

o **Eliminate Your Triggers**

Determine the primary sources of anxiety in your life. Is it your work, your travel, or your homework that is the problem? If you can figure out what they are, try if you can remove or at least lessen them from your life.

Chapter 9: Easy Healthy and Delicious Recipes

There are a variety of dishes here that will suit excellently with your new IF regimen. They include classics including Bacon, Vegetable Omelet, Scrambler, and Lemon Thyme Chicken, as well as conventional and vegetarian options. Every meal is covered, from breakfast to supper, with soup, salad, and snacks in between. Desserts like Peach Tart and Peanut Butter Cookies, of course, are always nice. You will undoubtedly enjoy yourself while preparing these delectable dinners.

9.1. Recipes for Breakfast

9.1.1. Vanilla Cinnamon Pancake

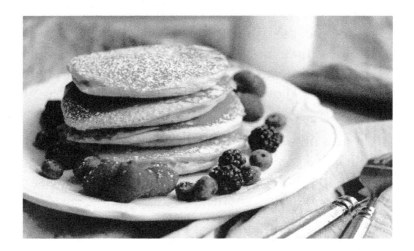

- o Preparation Time: 10 minutes
- o Cooking Time: 20 minutes
- o Total Time: 30 minutes
- o Servings: 2 (six pancakes)

The **ingredients** are as follows:

- o 2 eggs, large
- o 2/3 cup almond flour (blanched)
- o 2 ounces (56 g) softened cream cheese
- o 2 tsp vanilla extract (pure)
- o 1 tbsp stevia or monk fruit flakes
- o 1 tbsp baking soda
- o 1/2 tsp cinnamon powder
- o sea salt, to taste
- o butter, berries, and full-fat yogurt (optional)

- **Directions**

  - o Combine the vanilla, stevia, baking powder, almond flour, cinnamon, eggs, cream cheese, and salt in the container of a food blender. Blend until completely smooth. Allow 5 minutes for the sauce to thicken slightly.

  - o Heat a non-stick griddle pan over moderate heat lightly oiled. To create six pancakes, drop a scant 3 tbsp batter onto the skillet for each one. Cook for 2 minutes or until surface bubbles emerge.

  - o Turn the pancakes over with care. Cook for 1 minute, until golden brown.

- o Serve the pancakes with butter, berries, and yogurt right away (if using).

- **Nutritional fact:**384 calories. 34 grams of fat. 16 grams of carbohydrates. 15 grams of protein. 3 grams of fiber.

9.1.2. Apple Cinnamon Oatmeal

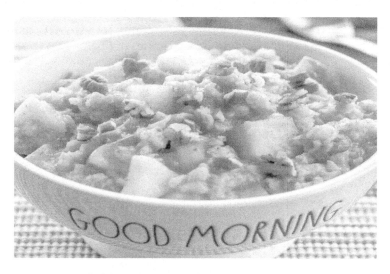

- o Preparation Time: 5 minutes

- o Cooking Time: 15 minutes

- o Total Time: 20 minutes

- o Servings: 2

The **ingredients** are as follows:

- o 1 cup oats

- o 1 apple, peeled and sliced into bite-size portions

- o 1 3/4 cup water

- o 1 tsp maple nectar

- o 1 tsp of cinnamon

- **Directions**

    o 1 3/4 cup water, oatmeal, and cinnamon, brought to a boil, then reduced to low heat and frequently stirred until it thickens.

    o Mix in the maple nectar well, then divide over two bowls and garnish with apples.

- **Nutritional fact:** 129 calories. 1.5 grams of fat. 27 grams of carbohydrates. 3 grams of protein. 25 grams of fiber.

9.1.3. Healthy Chia and Oats Smoothie

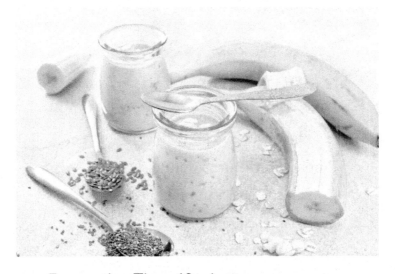

    o Preparation Time: 10 minutes

    o Cooking Time: 0 minutes

    o Total Time: 10 minutes

    o Servings: 2

The **ingredients** are as follows:

    o 1 cup of almond milk

    o 2 tbsp chia seeds

o   12 bananas (chopped)

o   6 tbsp oats

o   2 tbsp hemp seeds

o   4 dates (optional)

Directions

o   In a blender, combine all the ingredients and mix until smooth.

o   Pour into glasses and serve immediately.

- **Nutritional fact:** 140 calories. 7 grams of fat. 12 grams of carbohydrates. 12 grams of protein. 4 grams of fiber.

9.1.4. Ham & Veggie Omelet

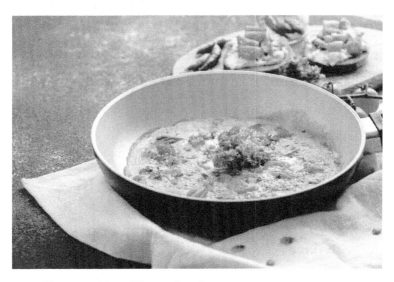

o   Preparation Time: 2 minutes

o   Cooking Time: 10 minutes

o   Total Time: 12 minutes

o   Servings: 2

The **ingredients** (for Ham Omelet) are as follows:

- o   2 eggs (large)
- o   2 tbsp cheese (feta, sharp cheddar, or goat cheese)
- o   2 tbsp diced ham
- o   4 cherry tomatoes, quartered
- o   1 tbsp red onion, diced
- o   Olive oil spray
- o   Salt and pepper

The **ingredients** (for Vegetarian Omelet) are as follows:

- o   3 eggs (large)
- o   2 tbsp cheese (feta, sharp cheddar, or goat cheese)
- o   2 tbsp mushrooms (sliced)
- o   1/8 cup baby spinach
- o   5 cherry tomatoes, quartered
- o   2 tbsp red onion, diced
- o   Salt and pepper
- o   Olive oil spray

- **Directions**

  - o   Place a small skillet over medium heat, lightly sprayed with olive oil spray.
  - o   Whisk together the eggs, one teaspoon of water, and a sprinkle of salt and pepper in a medium mixing bowl.
  - o   Add the eggs in the heated skillet and cook, occasionally stirring, until they begin to boil and break away from the pan's edges.

o On one half of the omelet, spread 1/2 of the cheese, then top with vegetables, ham (if using) and the remaining cheese.

o Heat for 2 minutes after folding the bare half over the half with the contents.

o Before transferring to a dish, turn and cook for another 2 minutes. Serve immediately.

- **Nutritional fact:** 232 calories. 15.3 grams of fat. 6.4 grams of carbohydrates. 17.6 grams of protein. 1.4 grams of fiber.

9.1.5. Herb Scramble with Spicy Tomatoes and Mushrooms

o Preparation Time: 5 minutes

o Cooking Time: 8 minutes

o Total Time: 13 minutes

o Servings: 2

The **ingredients** are as follows:

o 4 eggs (large)

o 1 tbsp butter

o 2 tbsp heavy cream

o ¼ cup grated white Cheddar cheese

o 1 tbsp chopped dill, with additional sprigs for garnish

o 1 tbsp chopped flat-leaf parsley

o Sea salt, to taste

o Serve with microgreens (optional)

The **ingredients** (Spicy tomatoes and mushrooms) are as follows:

- o 1 tbsp butter
- o 6 ounces (170g) grape or cherry tomatoes
- o 6 ounces (170g) quartered brown mushrooms
- o Freshly ground black pepper, to taste
- o Sea salt, to taste
- o Pinch of crushed red pepper

- **Directions**

  - o To prepare the chili tomatoes, and mushrooms, combine all the ingredients in a large mixing bowl. Melt the butter in a medium or large pan over medium-high heat. Combine the mushrooms and tomatoes in a mixing bowl. Cook, stirring periodically, for approximately 5 minutes, or until the tomatoes are roasted as well as the mushrooms are browned.

  - o Combine the chopped red pepper, salt, and pepper in a mixing bowl. Cook, constantly stirring until everything is well mixed.

  - o Prepare the eggs while the mushrooms and tomatoes are frying. Melt the butter in a small non-stick pan over medium-low heat.

  - o Scramble eggs, parsley, cream, dill, and salt in a medium mixing bowl. Pour the mixture into the skillet. Cheddar cheese should be strewn over the eggs. Cook for 3 minutes, or until nearly set, stirring periodically. Remove the pan from the heat and gently fold the egg until it is barely done.

- o Serve the eggs with the tomato sauce, additional microgreens, and dill sprigs as soon as possible (if using).

- **Nutritional fact**369 calories. 30 grams of fat. 8 grams of carbohydrates. 18 grams of protein. 1 gram of fiber.

9.1.6. Tomato Baked Eggs

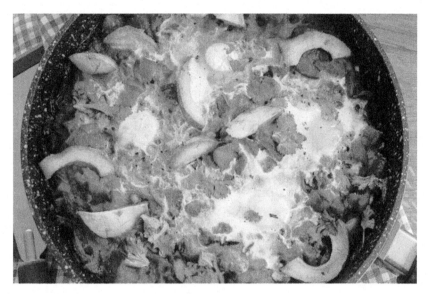

- o Preparation Time: 15 minutes
- o Cooking Time: 25 minutes
- o Total Time: 40 minutes
- o Servings: 2

The **ingredients** are as follows:

- o 4 eggs (large)
- o 1 sliced avocado
- o 2 tbsp tomato paste
- o ½ cup red onion (diced)

- ½ cup diced red bell pepper (diced)
- 1 cup kale leaves (torn)
- 1½ tbsp avocado oil
- 2 garlic cloves, minced
- 2 tbsp coarsely cilantro, finely chopped
- 1 tsp paprika, smoked
- ¼ tsp cumin powder
- 1 (14 ounces/396g) can fire-roasted diced tomatoes, undrained
- 2 tsp harissa paste (a North African chili paste, or use a pinch of crushed red pepper)
- 1/3 cup crumbled feta cheese, or another favorite cheese such as Parmesan, Cheddar, or smoked Gouda
- Sea salt and black pepper, to taste

- **Directions**

  - Preheat the microwave to 375 degrees Fahrenheit (190 degrees Celsius). Heat the oil using a large oven-safe pan over medium heat. Combine the onions, garlic, and bell pepper in a mixing bowl. Cook for 5 minutes, or until the pepper and onion are softened, stirring periodically.
  - Combine the harissa, tomato paste, cumin, and paprika in a mixing bowl. Cook for 30 seconds, stirring constantly, or until aromatic.
  - Add the tomatoes and their juices, as well as the salt and pepper. Cook, uncovered, for 5 - 6 minutes or until the gravy thickens, stirring periodically. Turn off the heat.
  - Make four indentations in the sauce, equally spaced, and break an egg into each. Arrange the kale surrounding the

eggs and along the skillet's border. Season with salt & pepper.

o Bake for 12 minutes or until the eggs become firm, but the yolks remain soft. Serve immediately with avocado, feta, and cilantro on top, directly from the pan.

- **Nutritional fact:** 330 calories. 20 grams of fat. 23 grams of carbohydrates. 16 grams of protein. 5 grams of fiber.

9.1.7. Mushroom and Asparagus Frittata

o Preparation Time: 15 minutes

o Cooking Time: 40 minutes

o Total Time: 55 minutes

o Servings: 2

The **ingredients** are as follows:

o 4 eggs (large)

o 2 tbsp cream or milk

o 1 tsp of butter

o 1/3 cup ricotta cheese

o 8 ounces (226g) small brown mushrooms, sliced

o ½ cup (0.5o ounces/14g) finely grated fresh Parmesan cheese

o 4 ounces (113g) asparagus, trimmed of woody ends and halved crosswise

o Sea salt and freshly ground black pepper, to taste

o 1 cup cherry tomatoes, halved, for serving

o 2 tbsp chopped basil, plus extra leaves for serving

- **Directions**

  o Preheat oven to 350 degrees Fahrenheit (180 degrees Celsius). Bring a medium pot with water to boil, then lower the heat to maintain a low simmer. Simmer the asparagus in a pan of water. Cook for 1 min, or until the color changes to a vivid green. Place the chicken on a platter lined with paper towels.

  o Over medium-high heat, melt the butter in a medium oven-safe non - stick frying pan (6–8in/15–20cm). Cook the mushroom in two batches for approximately 5 minutes, or until they have softened. Take the pan out of the oven. Clean the pan and brush it with a little additional butter on the bottom and sides.

  o Whisk the eggs, salt, milk, and pepper together in a medium bowl. Combine the Parmesan cheese, basil, and mushrooms in a large mixing bowl. To blend everything, whisk it together.

  o Fill the pan with the mixture carefully. Spread the asparagus within the egg mixture, then top with ricotta. Bake for 30 minutes, with the pan uncovered in the oven. Remove the pan from the heat and set it aside to cool. (The frittata may be served in the pan or pushed onto a dish.)

  o Extra basil leaves may be added to the top if desired. Make two wedges out of the potato. Using tomatoes on the side, serve warm or cold.

- **Nutritional fact:** 381 calories. 25 grams of fat. 13 grams of carbohydrates. 32 grams of protein. 3 grams of fiber.

9.1.8. Berry Prune Juice Smoothie

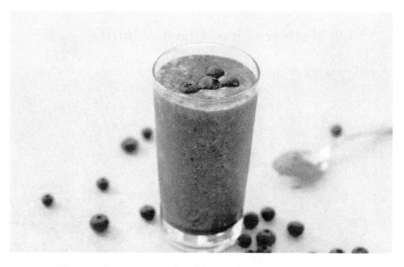

- o Preparation Time: 3 minutes
- o Cooking Time: 0 minutes
- o Total Time: 3 minutes
- o Servings: 2

The **ingredients** are as follows:

- o 1/2 cup coconut milk
- o 1/2 cup frozen blueberries
- o 1 tbsp chia seeds
- o 3/4 cups of ice
- o 1 cup Sunsweet Amazin Prune Juice
- o 1/2 cup spinach

- **Directions**

- o In a blender, combine all ingredients and mix until smooth.

- **Nutritional fact:** 252 calories. 14.2 grams of fat. 31.2 grams of carbohydrates. 3.4 grams of protein. 4.5 grams of fiber.

9.1.9. Blueberry Lime Almond Muffins

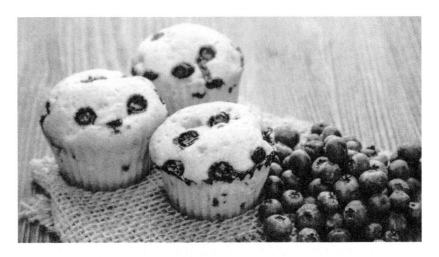

- o Preparation Time: 10 minutes
- o Cooking Time: 25 minutes
- o Total Time: 35 minutes
- o Servings: 12 muffins

The **ingredients** are as follows:

- o 1 cup milk (whole or almond)
- o 2 eggs (large)
- o 1 cup blueberries
- o ¼ cup coconut flour
- o 2 tbsp baking powder
- o 3 cups almond flour (blanched)
- o ½ tsp xanthan gum
- o 1 tsp pure vanilla extract

- o ½ cup avocado oil or melted butter
- o ½ tsp baking soda
- o 2 tbsp finely grated lime zest
- o 1⁄3 cup stevia or granulated monk fruit sweetener
- o Sea salt, to taste
- o Sliced almonds for topping (optional)

- **Directions**

  - o Preheat oven to 375 degrees Fahrenheit (190 degrees Celsius). Using cupcake liners, prepare a 12-cup muffin tray.

  - o Combine the coconut flour, almond flour, baking powder, baking soda, stevia, xanthan gum, and salt in a large mixing bowl and whisk until well blended.

  - o Stir in the blueberries with flour mixture until everything is well combined.

  - o Whisk the milk, eggs, oil, vanilla, and zest together in a medium mixing basin. Combine the flour and milk in a mixing bowl. Combine the ingredients in a small mixing bowl and stir until they are evenly distributed.

  - o Fill muffin cups three-quarters filled with the batter. (You can do this with an ice cream scoop.) Add the sliced almonds as a final touch (if using).

  - o Bake for 25 minutes, or until a toothpick placed in the middle comes out clean. Remove the muffins to a cooling rack after 5 minutes in the pan. Warm or room temperature are also acceptable serving options.

- **Nutritional fact:** 282 calories. 25 grams of fat. 11 grams of carbohydrates. 8 grams of protein. 4 grams of fiber.

9.1.10. Strawberry Shortcake Yogurt Bowls

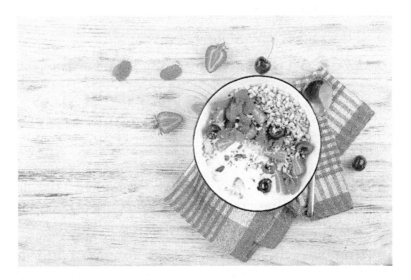

- o Preparation Time: 10 minutes
- o Cooking Time: 40 minutes
- o Total Time: 50 minutes
- o Serving: 3

The **ingredients** (Shortcake Granola) are as follows:

- o 1/2 cup olive oil
- o 3 cups rolled oats
- o 1 cup unsweetened coconut flakes, chopped
- o 1 cup sliced almonds
- o 3–4 tbsp turbinado sugar
- o 1 cup chopped pecans
- o 1 1/2 tsp vanilla
- o 1/2 cup pure maple syrup
- o 1 1/2 tsp salt

The **ingredients** (Yogurt Bowl Toppers) are as follows:

- o fresh strawberries
- o Siggi's triple cream vanilla yogurt
- o a pinch of sugar

- **Directions**

  - o Preheat the oven to 350°F for the granola. Mix everything together, including two teaspoons of turbinado sugar. Using a large non-stick baking pan, spread the mixture out. Bake for twenty minutes. Cook for another twenty minutes after stirring. Remove the turbinado sugar and stir with the remaining sugar. Allow to cool and crisp up in the pan.

  - o Strawberries should be cut into tiny pieces. To make them juicier, mash them a little with a fork. Add a smidgeon of more white or raw sugar. Voilà, strawberries that have been macerated.

  - o Bowls: Toss the Siggi's yogurt with a handful of granola and strawberries in a bowl. It is delicious.

- **Nutritional fact:** 339 calories. 22.4 grams of fat. 29.9 grams of carbohydrates. 5.2 grams of protein. 4.4 grams of fiber.

9.2. Recipes for Lunch

9.2.1. Salmon and kale frittata

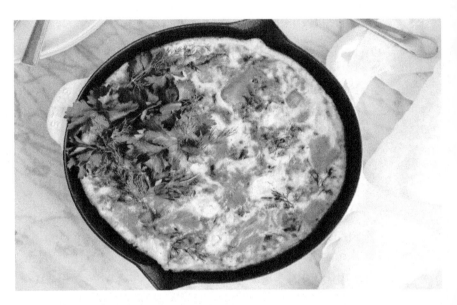

- o Preparation Time: 10 minutes
- o Cooking Time: 25 minutes
- o Total Time: 35 minutes
- o Servings: 2

The **ingredients** are as follows:

- o 6 eggs (large)
- o 4 ounces (113g) cooked skin-off salmon, flaked
- o 1 tbsp avocado oil
- o ½ cup ricotta cheese
- o ½ cup heavy whipping cream
- o 1/3 cup white cheddar cheese, grated

- o 2 cups (2ounces/60g) kale leaves, shredded
- o 2 tbsp chopped dill, plus extra for garnish
- o Pinch of nutmeg, grounded
- o Sea salt, to taste
- o black pepper, to taste

- **Directions**

  - o Preheat the microwave to 400 degrees Fahrenheit (200 degrees Celsius). Mix together the cream, eggs, nutmeg, dill, salt, and pepper in a medium mixing basin.

  - o Over medium heat, heat an 8-inch (20-cm) non-stick oven-safe skillet. Swirl in the oil to coat the skillet's bottom and sides.

  - o Cook for 2 - 3 mins or until the kale is barely wilted.

  - o Toss the fish into the pan. Pour the egg mixture into the pan, stirring it around to ensure that it is equally distributed. Place the ricotta on top of the ricotta mixture. Cheddar cheese should be sprinkled on top. Reduce heat to a low setting. Cook for 7 minutes, uncovered.

  - o Bake for 15 minutes in an uncovered pan in the oven. Allow cooling completely in the pan. (You may serve the frittata in the pan or transfer it onto a platter.)

  - o Add more dill if desired. Cut each wedge into three pieces and serve.

Nutritional fact: 498 calories. 40 grams of fat. 7 grams of carbohydrates. 29 grams of protein. 1 gram of fiber.

9.2.2. Grilled Green Goodness Salad

- o Preparation Time: 20 minutes
- o Cooking Time: 13 minutes
- o Total Time: 33 minutes
- o Servings: 2

The **ingredients** are as follows:

- o 6 ounces (170g) skin-on salmon fillet
- o 2 tbsp sunflower seeds, raw
- o 1 ½ cup strawberries (hulled), sliced
- o 5 ounces (141g) sugar snap peas, trimmed
- o 2 tsp avocado oil, divided
- o 5 ounces (142g) broccoli florets (about 2 cups)
- o 10 asparagus spears, trimmed of woody ends
- o 4 scallions, thinly sliced
- o 4 cups baby spinach leaves
- o Sea salt, to taste
- o black pepper, to taste

The **ingredients** (Cilantro-lime dressing) are as follows:

- o 1 garlic clove
- o 3 tbsp lime juice, fresh
- o 2 tbsp avocado oil
- o 1 tsp coconut aminos
- o 3 tbsp cilantro, chopped
- o 1 tsp Dijon mustard

o Pinch of granulated monk or stevia fruit sweetener (optional)

- **Directions**

o To make the cilantro-lime dressing, combine all the ingredients in a mixing bowl and whisk to combine until smooth blend. Put it in the fridge until you are ready to use it.

o Prepare a grill or grill pan to moderate temperatures. Using a knife, cut the fish in half. Each fillet should be brushed with 12 teaspoons of oil. Using salt & pepper, season to taste. Cook for 3 minutes with the salmon skin side down. Cook for another 2 minutes. (Cooking time varies according to fillet thickness.) Remove the heat from the room. Remove the salmon skin, flake it up, and put it aside.

o 1/2 inch (1.25 cm) thick pieces of broccoli, cut lengthwise.

o Toss the broccoli, asparagus, one teaspoon oil, sugar snap peas, and salt & pepper in a large mixing basin until the veggies are well covered in oil. Cook for two to four minutes on each side on the grill, in batches, until grill marks develop, and the veggies are tender-crisp. Allow cooling completely before serving. If desired, shred the broccoli.

o Divide the spinach into two serving dishes, then top with the grilled veggies, flakes salmon, and dressing. Strawberries are added last. Add the onions and sunflower seeds and toss to combine. Right away, serve.

- **Nutritional fact:** 477 calories. 30 grams of fat. 31 grams of carbohydrates. 27 grams of protein. 10 grams of fiber

9.2.3. Butter Chicken

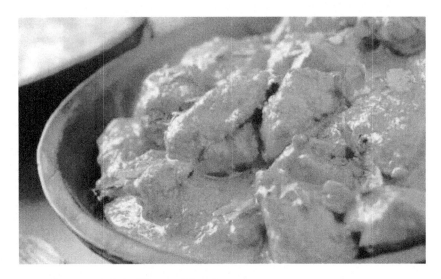

- o Preparation Time: 10 minutes
- o Cooking Time: 15 minutes
- o Total Time: 25 minutes
- o Servings: 2

The **ingredients** (for the marinated chicken) are as follows:

- o 1 lb. skinless, boneless, skinless chicken breasts (cut into 1-inch cubes)
- o 2 tbsp plain Greek yogurt
- o 1/2 tsp x ginger, grounded
- o 1/2 tbsp lemon juice
- o 2 tbsp tomato paste
- o 1/4 tsp turmeric
- o 1 tsp garam masala
- o 1/2 tsp ground coriander
- o 2 tbsp cayenne pepper

- o 1 tsp cumin
- o 3/8 tsp freshly ground black pepper
- o 1/4 tsp cinnamon
- o 1/2 tsp salt

The **ingredients** (for cooking) are as follows:

- o 1/4 cup plain Greek yogurt
- o 1/2 small onion, diced
- o 2.5 cloves garlic, minced
- o 1/2 tbsp canola oil
- o 21 tbsp light brown sugar
- o 1/4 cup water

- **Directions**

  - o In a dish or a tiptop plastic bag, place the sliced chicken pieces. In a mixing dish, mix all the marinade ingredients and toss thoroughly. (It will be rather thick.) Pour the marinade mixture over the meat and toss to evenly coat. Allow for a minimum of 30 mins. And up to eight hours of marinating time (see notes).

  - o In a large skillet, heat the oil over medium-high heat. Canola oil should be added at this point.

  - o Cook for 2-3 mins. or until onion is softened. Cook for a further minute after adding the garlic.

  - o Toss the marinated chicken into the pan. Cook for 2-3 mins. After adding the brown sugar.

  - o Reduce heat to moderate or medium-low to maintain a consistent simmer after adding the yogurt and water. Allow for another 8-10 minutes of cooking time, or until the meat is cooked through and the sauce has thickened.

o   Season with salt & pepper to taste.

o   Serve it hot with a dollop of additional sauce on top.

- **Nutritional fact:** 327 calories. 7 grams of fat. 10 grams of carbohydrates. 51 grams of protein. 1 gram of fiber.

9.2.4. Creamy Mushroom Soup

o   Preparation Time: 15 minutes

o   Cooking Time: 23 minutes

o   Total Time: 38 minutes

o   Servings: 2

The **ingredients** are as follows:

o   1/2 tbsp butter

o   6 tbsp heavy cream

o   2 garlic cloves, minced

o   2.5 cups chicken or vegetable broth

o   1 /2 tbsp avocado oil

o   1 lb. mixed mushrooms, sliced

o   1/2 cup sliced scallions, plus extra for garnish

o   1/4 cup dry sherry or dry white wine

o   1/2 tsp sea salt

o   1 /2 tsp freshly ground black pepper

o   Pinch of nutmeg, grounded

o   1/4 tsp xanthan gum Sour cream (optional) for serving

o   2 Garlic Rolls, for serving

- **Directions**

  o Melt the butter and oil in a Dutch oven or heavy-bottomed stockpot over medium-high heat. Combine the scallions, garlic, and mushrooms in a large mixing bowl.

  o Cook, uncovered, for 5 to 7 minutes, stirring occasionally.

  o Combine the pepper, salt, sherry, and nutmeg in a mixing bowl. Cook for 1 minute, stirring constantly.

  o Pour in the broth. Bring to a boil, then lower to a low heat setting. Cover and cook for 10 minutes. Toss in the thick cream and whisk well. Allow 5 minutes for cooling.

  o Pour the soup into a mixer in 2 or 3 batches and mix until completely smooth. Put the mixture back in the same pot. (Alternatively, mix straight in the saucepan using an immersion blender.)

  o Xanthan gum should be added now. Over medium heat, whisk until the soup is heated and thickened. If the soup gets too thick, add additional broth.

  o Individual pieces should be served right away with a tablespoon of thick cream (if used) and 1/2 of a roll for dipping.

- **Nutritional fact:** 314 calories. 24 grams of fat. 14 grams of carbohydrates. 10 grams of protein. 3 grams of fiber.

9.2.5. Waffles Made with Greek Chickpeas

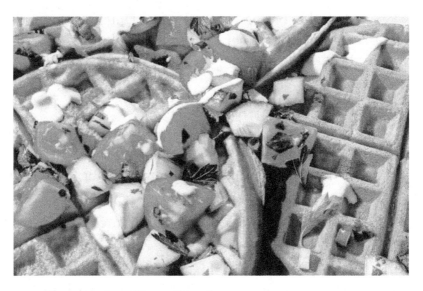

- o Preparation Time: 20 minutes
- o Cooking Time: 10 minutes
- o Total Time: 35 minutes
- o Servings: 2

The **ingredients** are as follows:

- o 6 eggs (large)
- o ¾ cup plain Greek yogurt
- o ¾ cup chickpea flour
- o ½ tsp baking soda
- o Tomatoes, parsley, cucumbers, lemon juice, olive oil, scallion, and yogurt for serving
- o ½ tsp salt
- o black pepper, to taste

- **Directions**

  - Heat the microwave to around 200 degrees Fahrenheit (180 degrees Celsius) and arrange a wire rack over a baking tray. The waffle iron should be preheated according to the manufacturer's instructions.

  - Combine baking soda, salt, and flour in a large mixing basin. Combine the eggs and yogurt in a small mixing dish. Combine the wet and dry ingredients and mix well.

  - Using non-stick cooking spray, gently cover the waffle with a light coating. Drop 1/4 to 1/2 cup mixture into each part of the iron in batches and bake for 4 - 5 minutes, or until golden brown. Waffles should be kept warm in the oven. Replace the batter and repeat the process.

  - The flavorful tomato mixture may be served with the waffles or with a sprinkle of warm berries and nut butter.

- **Nutritional fact:** 412 calories. 18 grams of fat. 24 grams of carbohydrates. 35 grams of protein. 4 grams of fiber.

9.2.6. Greek Meatballs with Chunky Tomato Sauce

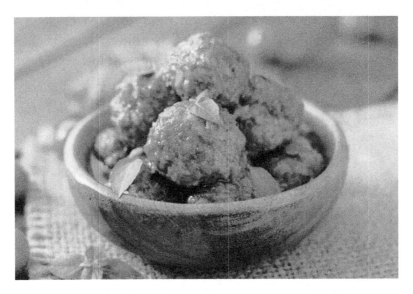

- o Preparation Time: 25 minutes
- o Cooking Time: 35 minutes
- o Total Time: 60 minutes
- o Servings: 2

The **ingredients** are as follows:

- o 1/2lb (225g) grounded beef (20% fat)
- o 1 tbsp olive oil
- o 2 garlic cloves, minced
- o 1/4 cup scallions, thinly sliced
- o 2 ounces (56.5g) crumbled feta cheese, plus extra for garnish
- o 1 tbsp chopped dill
- o 1/2 tbsp chopped oregano, plus extra for garnish
- o 1/2 tsp lemon zest, finely grated (optional)

- o 2 medium zucchinis, thinly sliced lengthwise

- o Sea salt, to taste

- o freshly ground black pepper, to taste

The **ingredients** (for Chunky tomato sauce) are as follows:

- o 1/2 cup beef or chicken broth

- o 1 tsp olive oil

- o 2 garlic cloves, minced

- o 1 tbsp tomato paste

- o 1/2 can (198g) fire-roasted diced tomatoes, undrained

- o 1/4 tsp red pepper, crushed

- o Sea salt, to taste

- o black pepper, to taste

- o Pinch of granulated monk or stevia fruit sweetener (optional)

- **Directions**

  - o To make the chunky tomato sauce, combine all of the ingredients in a mixing bowl. Warm the oil in a moderate skillet over medium heat. Cook for 1 min, or until garlic is fragrant. Add the broth, tomato with juices, crushed red pepper, tomato paste, salt, pepper, and stevia to the pot (if using). Bring to a boil, then turn down to low heat. Cook, uncovered, for 8 - 10 mins.

  - o Preheat the microwave to 375 degrees F (190 degrees C). Line a baking pan with foil. On the baking sheet, grease a wire rack.

  - o Combine the beef, garlic, scallions, dill, zest, oregano, feta, salt, and pepper in an intermediate bowl. Roll the dough into 24 balls with slightly damp palms to avoid sticking. Arrange the items on a wire rack. Bake for 22–25 minutes, or until golden brown and done.

o Put the zucchini in the oil while the meatballs cook. Season using salt & pepper to taste. Cook in stages on a heated grill pan until the zucchini is cooked and grill marks form.

o Serve the zucchini on four dishes. To serve, place six meatballs per dish, cover with sauce, and garnish with more feta and oregano leaves. Serve as soon as possible. Any leftover meatballs may be stored in an airtight jar in the freezer for up to five days or frozen for up to 3 months.

- **Nutritional fact:** 471 calories. 33 grams of fat. 17 grams of carbohydrates. 28 grams of protein. 4 grams of fiber.

9.2.7. Curried Chicken Salad

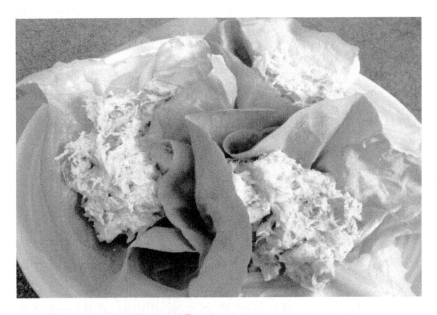

o Preparation Time: 15 minutes

o Cooking Time: 10 minutes

- o Total Time: 25 minutes
- o Servings: 2

The **ingredients** are as follows:

- o 2 tbsp olive oil
- o 8 ounces boneless, skinless chicken breast, cubed
- o 1 small yellow onion, diced
- o 1 stalk celery, sliced
- o 1/2 tsp curry powder
- o 4 cups baby romaine lettuce
- o 2 medium apples, chopped
- o 1/2 cup raw almonds, chopped
- o 1/2 English cucumber, diced

- **Directions**

  - o Cook the chicken, onion, and celery in olive oil for 10 minutes in a deep sauté pan over moderate heat. Allow 15 minutes for cooling.
  - o Mix almonds, cucumber, apples, and curry powder in a large mixing bowl with the cooled chicken mixture.
  - o Serve over a bed of baby romaine lettuce.

- **Nutritional fact:** 124 calories. 6.6 grams of fat. 8.1 grams of carbohydrates. 8.2 grams of protein. 2.4 grams of fiber.

9.2.8. Chicken Drumsticks Wrapped in Bacon

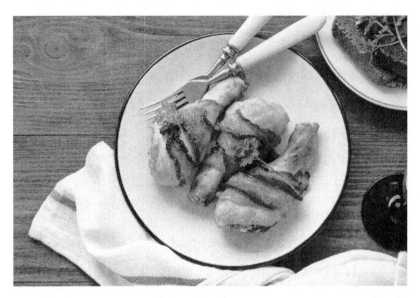

- o Preparation Time: 5 minutes
- o Cooking Time: 45 minutes
- o Total Time: 50 minutes
- o Servings: 2

The **ingredients** are as follows:

- o 4 portions of bacon, sliced
- o 4 chicken drumsticks
- o 1 tsp freshly ground black pepper
- o 1 ½ tsp Himalayan salt

- • **Directions**

- o Preheat oven to 400 degrees Fahrenheit (200 degrees Celsius). Wrap aluminum foil around a baking pan.

- o Working from the bottom to the top of the drumstick, wrap one slice of bacon over each one. Season with salt & pepper before placing on the preheated baking sheet.
- o Preheat the oven to 350°F and bake the bacon for approximately 45 minutes, or until crisp.

- **Nutritional fact:** 212.2 calories. 10.8 grams of fat. 4.8 grams of carbohydrates. 22.9 grams of protein. 0.6 grams of fiber.

9.2.9. Chicken Wraps

- o Preparation Time: 10 minutes
- o Cooking Time: 25 minutes
- o Total Time: 35 minutes
- o Servings: 2

The **ingredients** (for the chicken salad) are as follows:

- o 4.5 ounces (65 g) light cream cheese (11% fat)
- o 1 pound (450 g) chicken breast, skinless
- o 65 g Greek yogurt, low fat
- o 0.5 tsp chopped dill
- o 0.5 carrot
- o 0.25 tsp red wine vinegar
- o 0.5 tsp lemon juice, freshly squeezed

The **ingredients** (for the wraps) are as follows:

- o 2 whole-wheat tortillas
- o 0.25 small onion sliced
- o 6 thin sticks of cucumber
- o 6 thin slices of tomato
- o 1-1.5 crunchy lettuce leaves, chopped

- **Directions**

  o Boil the chicken breasts for 20-25 minutes at a low temperature. Allow cooling before serving.

  o Whip the cheese cream until it is totally soft in a small mixing bowl.

  o Whisk in the Greek yogurt until it is completely mixed.

  o Using a hand grater, shred the carrot and add it to the mixture.

  o Combine the chopped dill, vinegar, and fresh lemon juice in a mixing bowl. Salt & pepper to taste.

  o When the chicken is cold enough to handle, shred it and add it to the mixture.

  o Combine all of the ingredients well.

  o Two slices of tomato, a smidgeon of onion, two cucumber sticks, lettuce, and 1-2 tbsp of the chicken salad, wrapped in a wrap.

- **Nutritional fact:** 364.1 calories. 11.7 grams of fat. 29.3 grams of carbohydrates. 34.2 grams of protein. 3.8 grams of fiber.

9.2.10. Cauliflower Pizza Crust

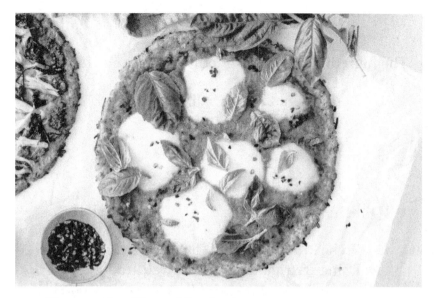

- o Preparation Time: 15 minutes
- o Cooking Time: 35 minutes
- o Total Time: 50 minutes
- o Servings: 2

The **ingredients** (for cauliflower pizza crust) are as follows:

- o 1 beaten egg
- o 1/4 cup shredded cheese
- o 1.5 pounds cauliflower florets
- o 1/2 tsp Italian seasoning
- o salt and pepper, to taste

The **ingredients** (for pesto chicken pizza) are as follows:

- o 1/4 cup shredded chicken
- o 2 garlic cloves, minced

- o 1/3 cup pesto sauce

- o 3/4 cup mozzarella cheese, shredded

- o 1 cup (packed) baby spinach

The **ingredients** (for Margherita pizza) are as follows:

- o 2 ounces mozzarella ball, sliced

- o 1/3 cup marinara sauce

- o fresh basil leaves

- o red pepper flakes (optional)

- **Directions**

  - o Preheat oven to 400° Fahrenheit (200 degrees Celsius). Using refrigerated & thawed cauliflower florets or removing the florets off the stalk Use a food blender or a box grater to grate the vegetables.

  - o Fill a microwave-safe bowl halfway with cauliflower rice, cover, and microwave for about 4-5 mins to soft. Alternatively, you may cook the cauliflower rice for 8-10 minutes in a pan over moderate heat on the stove. Allow it to cool completely before handling it.

  - o Fill a nut milk bag or a thin kitchen towel with the cauliflower rice. Squeeze the cauliflower until it is completely dry. Squeeze with all you might!

  - o In a large mixing dish, add the drained cauliflower rice. Season with salt, pepper, and cheese. To make the pizza dough, combine all ingredients with your hands.

  - o Squeeze the dough gently into a uniform circle on a parchment-lined baking pan. Around 9 inches in diameter is ideal. It is much better if you have a pizza pan since the crust will be crispier.

o Remove from the oven after 25 minutes of baking, or until brown. For an additional crispier crust, bake for 20 minutes, then turn the crust and bake for another 5-10 minutes.

o Bake for a further 10 minutes with the toppings on top.

- **Nutritional fact:** 177 calories. 11 grams of fat. 10 grams of carbohydrates. 13 grams of protein. 4 grams of fiber.

9.3. Recipes for Dinner

9.3.1. Roasted Cauliflower Rice

o Preparation Time: 10 minutes

o Cooking Time: 15 minutes

o Total Time: 25 minutes

o Servings: 2

The **ingredients** are as follows:

o 1 head cauliflower

o 1 cup rice

o ½ tsp Himalayan salt

o Herbs or spices (optional)

- **Directions**

o Preheat oven to 200 degrees Fahrenheit. Using parchment paper, line a baking sheet.

o Remove the stalks from the cauliflower and cut them into florets.

o Shred the cauliflower via hand or pulse it until it resembles rice in a food processor.

o Sprinkle the salt over the cauliflower rice upon this ready baking sheet.

o Preheat the oven to 350°F and bake the baking sheet for 12 -15 minutes, turning every 5 minutes. Remove the cauliflower rice before it begins to brown.

o Add any herbs or spices you like.

- **Nutritional fact:** 27 calories. 0.3 grams of fat. 5 grams of carbohydrates. 2 grams of protein. 2 grams of fiber.

9.3.2. Filet Mignon Salad

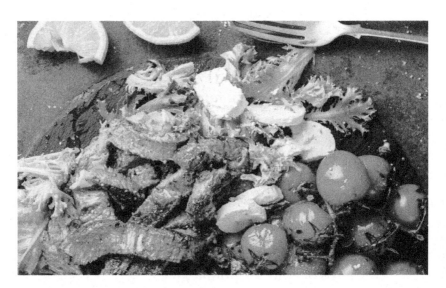

o Preparation Time: 12 minutes

o Cooking Time: 8 minutes

o Total Time: 20 minutes

o Servings: 2

The **ingredients** are as follows:

o 1/4 large head romaine lettuce, chopped and ribs removed

- o 8 cherry tomatoes, halved
- o 2 ounces goat cheese, crumbled
- o 1/2 large head (about 11/2 cups) Belgian endive trimmed and thinly sliced crosswise
- o 1 tbsp grass-fed butter, unsalted
- o 11/2 cups baby arugula
- o 1/4 cup fresh basil, chopped
- o 1/2-pound filet mignon
- o 1/2 cup plus
- o 1/2 cup rice wine vinegar
- o 11/2 tsp olive oil, divided
- o 11/2 tbsp lemon juice, freshly squeezed
- o 1/2 tsp freshly ground black pepper
- o 2 tsp pure maple syrup
- o 1/2 tsp sea salt

- **Directions**

  - o Add basil, romaine, endive, and arugula inside a large salad dish.

  - o Insert lemon juice, salt, maple syrup, vinegar, and pepper into a blender or food processor. Slowly drizzle in 1/2 cup oil while the machine is operating at low speed. Remove from the equation.

  - o One minute over medium heat, melt the butter with residual olive oil in an intermediate cast-iron or stainless-steel pan. Cook for 7 minutes on each side for moderate fillet mignon. Remove from the heat and set aside for 5 minutes. Cut the slices into medium-thick strips.

o   In a salad dish, combine the goat cheese, fillet mignon, and cherry tomatoes. The dressing should be added now. Serve after a good tossing to coat.

- **Nutritional fact:** 910 calories. 77.1 grams of fat. 12.7 grams of carbohydrates. 36.6 grams of protein. 4.1 grams of fiber.

9.3.3. Spinach and Feta-Stuffed Chicken Breasts

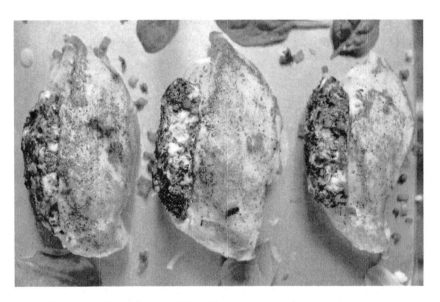

o   Preparation Time: 15 minutes

o   Cooking Time: 45 minutes

o   Total Time: 60 minutes

o   Servings: 2

The **ingredients** are as follows:

o   1 beaten egg (large)

o   2 (4-ounce) boneless, skinless chicken breasts, pounded to 1/4" thickness

o   1/2 cup crumbled feta cheese

- o 1 tbsp olive oil, garlic-infused
- o 1 cup fresh spinach leaves
- o 1 cup almond meal

- **Directions**

  - o Preheat the oven to 350 degrees Fahrenheit.

  - o One minute over low heat, heat the oil in an intermediate skillet. Cook for 3 minutes or until spinach is tender. Remove from heat after adding the feta and stirring a few times.

  - o Half of the spinach mixture should be placed on each chicken. Using toothpicks, secure the chicken around the mixture.

  - o Add the egg to a small basin. Almond grain should be placed in a separate shallow basin. Dip each breast in the egg, tapping out any excess, and then in the almond meal until thoroughly coated.

  - o In an 8" x 8" casserole dish, place the chicken. Bake for 30 minutes before serving.

- **Nutritional fact:** 395 calories. 24.1 grams of fat. 5.2 grams of carbohydrates. 35.8 grams of protein. 1.8 grams of fiber.

9.3.4. Red Chicken Curry with Zucchini Noodles

- o Preparation Time: 20 minutes
- o Cooking Time: 15 minutes
- o Total Time: 35 minutes
- o Servings: 2

The **ingredients** are as follows:

- o 1 cup (250ml) full-fat coconut milk

- o 2 small zucchinis (about 10 ounces/284g total)
- o 1 cup chicken broth
- o 6 ounces (170g) boneless skinless chicken thighs, chopped
- o 2-3 tbsp red curry paste
- o 1 tsp avocado oil
- o 2 tbsp coconut aminos
- o 2 tbsp lime juice. Freshly squeezed
- o 1/3 cup bean sprouts or pea shoots
- o 1/3 cup whole cilantro or Thai basil leaves, plus extra leaves for garnish
- o Thinly sliced scallions (optional)
- o garnish Lime wedges for serving

- **Directions**

  - o Remove the zucchini's ends and throw them away. To make zucchini strands that look like noodles, use a peeler. (This recipe yields about 4 cups.) Remove the item from circulation.

  - o Combine the curry paste, coconut aminos, coconut milk, and broth in a large sauté pan or wok (to taste). Bring to a boil over high heat, partly covered, then lower to medium. Cook for 10 minutes, uncovered.

  - o Meanwhile, heat the oil in a big pan over medium heat while the meat is frying. Combine the zucchini noodles with the other ingredients. Cook for 2 minutes, gently tossing occasionally.

  - o Toss the noodle mixture with lemon juice and cilantro. Combine all ingredients and stir well. In heated bowls, place the noodles. Over the noodles, ladle the curry.

o Serve with lime wedges and more cilantro, bean sprouts, and scallions (if using). Right away, serve.

- **Nutritional fact:** 424 calories. 32 grams of fat. 15 grams of carbohydrates. 22 grams of protein. 3 grams of fiber.

9.3.5. Sheet Pan Steak

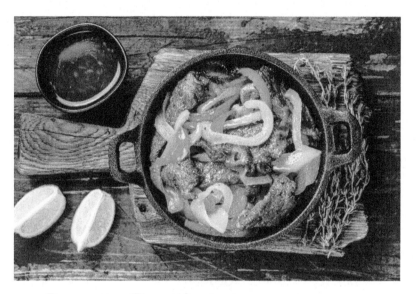

o Preparation Time: 13 minutes

o Cooking Time: 15 minutes

o Total Time: 28 minutes

o Servings: 2

The **ingredients** (for the fajitas) are as follows:

o 6 ounces flank steak, sliced into 1/4" strips across the grain

o 0.75 tbsp fresh cilantro, finely chopped

o juice from 2 limes, divided

o 2 medium bell peppers, thinly sliced

o   0.5 medium red onion, thinly sliced

o   1.5 tbsp olive oil divided

o   0.25 tsp Worcestershire sauce

The **ingredients** (for seasonings) are as follows:

o   0.5 tsp smoked paprika

o   0.5 tsp garlic powder

o   1 tsp chili powder

o   0.06 tsp cayenne pepper (optional), to taste

o   0.5 tsp cumin

o   0.25 - 0.5 tsp sea salt, to taste

The **ingredients** (for serving) as follows:

o   lime wedges

o   avocado, sliced

o   fresh cilantro, chopped

o   paleo / whole 30 tortillas

- **Directions**

  o   Preheat the oven to 400° degrees Fahrenheit and oil a baking sheet with cooking spray. You may also use parchment or foil to make cleaning simpler.

  o   In a small dish or bag, combine together the seasoning ingredients.

  o   Drizzle 1 1/2 teaspoons olive oil, one lime juice, Worcestershire sauce, and chopped cilantro over the steak in a big zip-top bag. Season with 2/3 of fajita spices. Toss well to coat. (For best taste, marinate for at least 30 minutes.

o On the prepared sheet pan, arrange the veggies in a uniform layer. Keep stuff in one layer, and don't overlap too much. (If required, use two sheet pans.) Drizzle the remaining 1 1/2 teaspoons olive oil over the top, then season with the remaining one-third (1/3) of the spices. Toss well to coat.

o Bake for 10-15 minutes or until peppers is soft in a preheated oven. (If the steak has been marinated in the fridge, take it from the fridge and set it aside to come to ambient temperature while the veggies are cooking.)

o Remove the sheet pan from the oven, turn it over, and press the veggies to the pan's edges. Place the steak pieces in one layer in the pan's middle, being careful not to overcrowd it. Broil for 3 minutes on high.

o Serve with chopped avocado and your preferred toppings on your favorite paleo/Whole30 tortillas.

o To bake tortillas, cover them in aluminum foil and place them on the top shelf of the oven for approximately 5 minutes while the chicken bakes.

- **Nutritional fact:** 266 calories. 15 grams of fat. 11 grams of carbohydrates. 20 grams of protein. 3 grams of fiber.

9.3.6. Spaghetti Bolognese

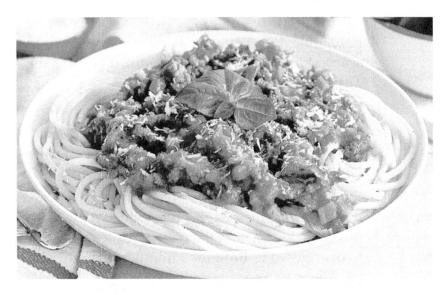

- o Preparation Time: 10 minutes
- o Cooking Time: 50 minutes
- o Total Time: 70 minutes
- o Servings: 2

The **ingredients** are as follows:

- o 150g dry spaghetti
- o 1/2 tbsp tomato puree
- o 1 onion, chopped
- o 1 clove garlic
- o 100g mushrooms
- o 3 sprays olive oil
- o 2 sticks celery
- o 2 carrots

- o 1/2 x 200g tomatoes, chopped
- o 1 /2 tsp dried oregano
- o 150g extra lean minced beef
- o 2 bay leaves

- **Directions**

  - o Slice the onions and mushrooms finely, celery and carrot finely, and garlic cloves.

  - o Using the oil, coat the bottom of a big non-stick pan with a lid. Stir in the mince after 5 minutes to break it up.

  - o Cook for another 5 minutes, stirring regularly.

  - o Combine the tomatoes, herbs, and tomato puree in a large mixing bowl.

  - o Cook for 40 mins, stirring periodically.

  - o Serve with spaghetti prepared according to package directions or to your preference.

  - o This sauce is much better the following day (refrigerate overnight) and freezes well.

- **Nutritional fact**457 calories. 9.2 grams of fat. 165.3 grams of carbohydrates. 28.8 grams of protein. 5.2 grams of fiber.

9.3.7. Baked Scallops

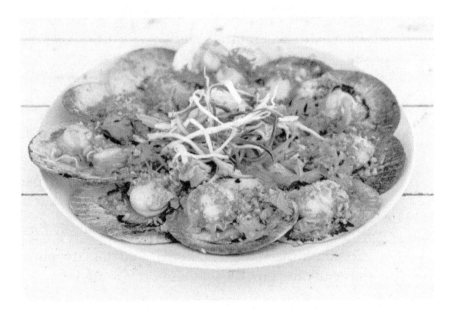

- o Preparation Time: 5 minutes
- o Cooking Time: 20 minutes
- o Total Time: 25 minutes
- o Servings: 2

The **ingredients** are as follows:

- o 2 tbs butter
- o 3 tbs Parmesan cheese, finely grated
- o ¼ tsp garlic powder
- o ½ tsp paprika
- o ½ lb. sea scallops (about 10-12)
- o fresh parsley, chopped (to garnish)
- o salt and black pepper, to taste
- o splash white wine, (optional)

- **Directions**

  o Preheat oven to 350 degrees Fahrenheit (180 degrees Celsius).

  o In a small mixing bowl, combine the Parmesan cheese, paprika, garlic powder, salt, and pepper.

  o Melt some butter in a medium baking dish and pour it into the bottom. If using, pour in the white wine in a baking dish, place the scallops.

  o Wrap in foil & roast for 20 mins or until the scallops have reached an internal body temperature of 125-130F.

  o Remove the foil and brown the tops for a few minutes on a warm broiler

  o Serve with a garnish of fresh parsley.

- **Nutritional fact:** 215 calories. 14 grams of fat. 4 grams of carbohydrates. 16 grams of protein. 0 grams of fiber.

9.3.8. Lamb Patties

  o Preparation Time: 5 minutes

  o Cooking Time: 15 minutes

  o Total Time: 20 minutes

  o Servings: 2

The **ingredients** are as follows:

  o 1 egg white

  o 1/2-pound ground lamb

  o 2 cloves garlic, peeled and minced

  o 1 medium shallot, peeled and minced

  o 1/4 cup dried currants

  o 1/2 tsp ground cinnamon

- o 1/4 cup whole pistachio nuts
- o 1/4 tsp black peppercorns, freshly cracked
- o 1/8 tsp salt

- **Directions**

  - o Preheat the oven to 350 degrees Fahrenheit.
  - o Combine shallots, garlic, lamb, egg, currants, almonds, and cinnamon in a mixing bowl. Season with salt & pepper.
  - o Make six little ovals out of the mixture. Bake for 15 minutes in an 8" x 8" baking dish. Serve warm.

- **Nutritional fact:** 399 calories. 21.8 grams of fat. 21.4 grams of carbohydrates. 27.3 grams of protein. 3.60 grams of fiber.

9.3.9. Chicken Burgers

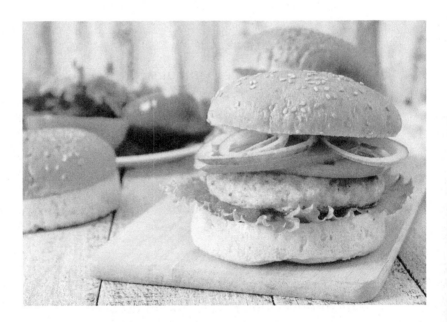

- o Preparation Time: 10 minutes
- o Cooking Time: 10 minutes
- o Total Time: 20 minutes
- o Servings: 2

The **ingredients** are as follows:

- o 0.5-pound chicken, grounded
- o 1 garlic clove, minced (or 1/2 tsp garlic powder)
- o 0.25 cup finely diced onion (or 1/2 tsp onion powder)
- o freshly ground black pepper
- o 0.38 tsp fine sea salt
- o 0.13 tsp smoked paprika (optional)

- **Directions**

  - o Mix the chicken, salt, onion, garlic, paprika, and a pinch of black pepper together in a large mixing basin. To make the patties, whisk everything together with a spoon, then split the mixture into four equal portions.

  - o Wet your hands to make the mixture better to handle (it does not adhere to wet palms) and press the mixture between your palms to create a burger patty. Rep with the remaining material until you have four 1-inch-thick patties.

  - o Place a 12-inch skillet over moderate heat on the stove and grease it with olive oil. Cook for 5 mins after arranging all four chicken burgers in the skillet. Cook for 5 - 6 minutes on the opposite side, or until a thermometer reads 165°F. (Alternatively, you can just chop one in half to ensure it is not pink in the center.)

  - o Warm-cooked burgers with your choice toppings are served. You may use a lettuce wrap or a bun! Cooked burgers may be stored in a sealed container in the refrigerator for up to three days or frozen for up to three months.

- **Nutritional fact:** 173 calories. 9 grams of fat. 2 grams of carbohydrates. 20 grams of protein. 1 gram of fiber.

9.3.10. One-Pan Prosciutto-Wrapped Shrimp and Broccoli

- o Preparation Time: 15 minutes
- o Cooking Time: 25 minutes
- o Total Time: 40 minutes
- o Servings: 2

The **ingredients** are as follows:

- o 2 tbsp olive oil, divided
- o 16 large raw shrimp, peeled and deveined, tails intact
- o 2 garlic cloves, sliced
- o 8 slices prosciutto, halved lengthwise
- o 2 tbsp flat-leaf parsley, chopped
- o 6 small bell peppers (any colors), halved, seeds and membranes removed
- o 16 ounces (487g) broccoli, trimmed and cut into florets
- o ½ tsp red pepper, crushed
- o 6 tbsp (42g) sliced almonds, toasted
- o Sea salt and black pepper, to taste
- o 1 lemon, sliced, plus extra wedges for serving

- **Directions**

  o Preheat the microwave to 400 degrees Fahrenheit (200 degrees Fahrenheit). Using parchment paper, line a baking sheet.

  o Toss lemon slices, 1 tbsp oil, bell pepper halves, broccoli, salt, and pepper on a baking sheet. 7 minutes of roasting

  o Each shrimp should be wrapped in half a piece of prosciutto. Toss the covered shrimp with the pepper and broccoli concoction that has been half-cooked. Drizzle the remaining 1 tbsp of oil on top. Add the crushed red pepper and garlic. Toss everything together. Bake for 15 minutes, or until the veggies are tender-crisp and the shrimp are almost done.

  o Toss in the parsley. Toss everything together. Serve warm with lemon wedges and a sprinkle of almonds.

- **Nutritional fact:** 512 calories. 363 grams of fat. 23 grams of carbohydrates. 28 grams of protein. 11 grams of fiber.

9.4. Additional Side Recipes

9.4.1. Almond Thyme Green Beans

- o Preparation Time: 10 minutes
- o Cooking Time: 6 minutes
- o Total Time: 16 minutes
- o Servings: 2

The **ingredients** are as follows:

- o ½ lb. (225g) green beans, stem ends removed
- o 1 tbsp butter
- o 1 garlic clove, minced
- o 1 tbsp sliced almonds, toasted
- o 1/2 tsp thyme, chopped (plus extra for garnish)
- o Pinch of red pepper, crushed
- o Sea salt, to taste

- **Directions**

  - o Boil or steam the beans in a large pot for 3 to 4 minutes, or until brilliant green and tender-crisp. Set aside the green beans after draining them in a colander.
  - o In the same pot, melt the butter. Cook for 30 seconds or until the garlic is aromatic.
  - o Combine the almonds, green beans, thyme, crushed red pepper, and salt in a large mixing bowl. Stir until everything is well blended. Arrange the ingredients on a serving plate. Serve immediately with additional thyme as a garnish.

- **Nutritional fact:** 59 calories. 4 grams of fat. 6 grams of carbohydrates. 2 grams of protein. 2 grams of fiber.

9.4.2. Mustard Rosemary Brussels Sprouts

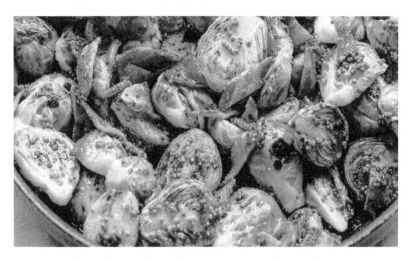

- o Preparation Time: 10 minutes
- o Cooking Time: 20 minutes
- o Total Time: 30 minutes
- o Servings: 2

The **ingredients** are as follows:

- o 1 lb. (450g) Brussels sprouts, trimmed and halved
- o 2 slices cooked bacon, diced
- o tbsp melted butter
- o ½ tsp garlic power
- o 1 tbsp Dijon mustard
- o ½ tsp chopped rosemary
- o 1 tbsp avocado oil

o 1 tsp granulated monk or stevia fruit sweetener (optional)

o ½ tsp sea salt, to taste

- **Directions**

  o Preheat the oven at 400 degrees Fahrenheit (200 degrees Celsius) before beginning. Use parchment paper to cover a baking pan.

  o Toss the butter, garlic powder, Brussels sprouts, oil, rosemary, salt, mustard, stevia, and bacon together in a large mixing basin.

  o Place Brussels sprouts cut side downwards on a baking sheet in a single layer. Roast for 15 - 20 minutes, or until tender-crisp and cooked through. Right away, serve.

- **Nutritional fact:**153 calories. 11 grams of fat. 10 grams of carbohydrates. 5 grams of protein. 4 grams of fiber.

9.4.3. Baked Chicken Wings

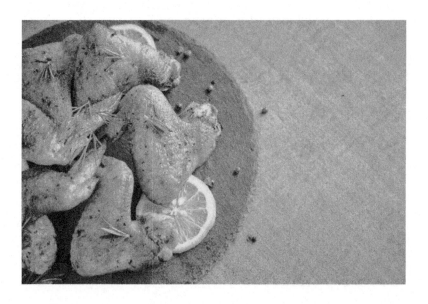

- o Preparation Time: 15 minutes
- o Cooking Time: 40 minutes
- o Total Time: 55 minutes
- o Servings: 2

The **ingredients** are as follows:

- o 1.5 lb. chicken wings, split, tips removed
- o 1 tbsp butter, melted
- o 0.5 tsp garlic powder
- o 0.5 tsp paprika (or smoked paprika)
- o 0.25 tsp black pepper
- o 1 tsp diamond crystal salt

- **Directions**

  - o Preheat the microwave to 400 degrees Fahrenheit (200 degrees Celsius). Use foil to line 2 rimmed baking sheets and wire racks to fit them.
  - o If your wings are entire, remove the tips & separate the drumettes from the flats
  - o Combine the chicken wings and melted butter in a large mixing basin.
  - o Place the coated chicken on the wire racks in a single layer, making sure they do not touch. Salt, garlic powder, and paprika should be sprinkled over the top.
  - o Cook the wings for approximately 40 minutes, or until the surface is golden brown and crispy.

- **Nutritional fact:** 380 calories. 25 grams of fat. 0.1 grams of carbohydrates. 35 grams of protein. 0.9 grams of fiber.

9.4.4. Cranberry Chutney

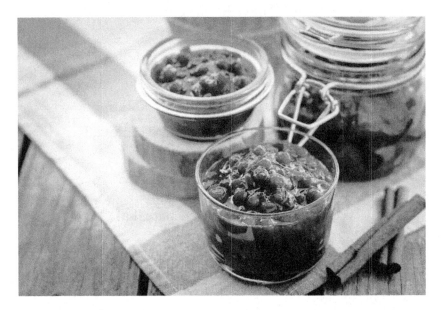

- o Preparation Time: 5 minutes
- o Cooking Time: 15 minutes
- o Total Time: 20 minutes
- o Servings: 2

The **ingredients** are as follows:

- o 2 cups fresh or frozen cranberries
- o 6 whole cloves
- o 1 cup coconut sugar
- o 1/4 cup red onion, peeled and finely diced

- **Directions**

  - o In a medium, heavy-bottomed saucepot, combine all of the ingredients. Simmer for 15 minutes on low heat or until all of the cranberries have broken down and the sauce has a saucy consistency. Remove the pan from the heat.

- **Nutritional fact:** 414 calories. 0.1 grams of fat. 110.1 grams of carbohydrates. 0.6 grams of protein. 4.9 grams of fiber.

9.4.5. Banana and Cacao Pudding

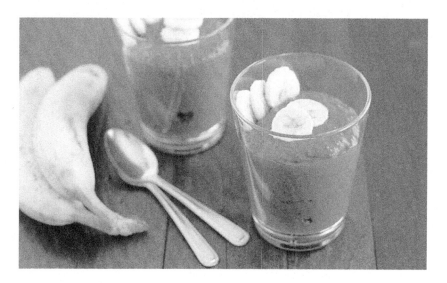

- o Preparation Time: 5 minutes
- o Cooking Time: 15 minutes
- o Total Time: 20 minutes
- o Servings: 2

The **ingredients** are as follows:

- o 1 tbsp coconut oil
- o 3 large ripe bananas, peeled
- o 1/8 tsp salt
- o 2 tbsp raw cacao powder, unsweetened

- **Directions**

  o Using a potato masher, mash bananas in a medium bowl. Mash in the coconut oil until everything is well combined.

  o Mix in the cacao powder well. Mix in the salt.

  o Serve alone or with a sauce for apple wedges.

- **Nutritional fact:** 260 calories. 7.3 grams of fat. 49.6 grams of carbohydrates. 3.2 grams of protein. 6.3 grams of fiber.

Chapter 10: Frequently Asked Questions (FAQs) About IF

The following are answers to some of the most frequently asked questions concerning intermittent fasting.

- **Is it Difficult to Stick to Intermittent Fasting?**

Some people may find it tough. You may face obstacles and problems, particularly if you are a novice and your body is still adjusting to the new habit and eating pattern. You will realize the eating schedule more manageable and simpler to follow after your body has adjusted.

The fundamental idea is to become more conscious of what and when you should consume. With such knowledge, you will be able to recognize the limits and constraints you must respect. It is also a good idea to combine this strategy with regular exercise and eating nutritious foods like fruits, beans, vegetables, healthy fats, lean meats, and lentils.

It is also important to stay away from too much salt and sugar. Sticking to IF will become less difficult after your body adjusts to these new rules.

- **What Is the Appropriate Fasting Duration in Hours/Days?**

The majority of IF practitioners adjust their fasting period to around16 hours every day. Most people follow this practice since it is simple to adapt and stick to. You may achieve it simply by missing breakfast the day following your last meal. If you are able, you may also try the IF diet, which asks you to stay without eating for 24 hours twice a week.

- **Is it Still Necessary for Me to Count Calories?**

The answer will be determined by the objectives you wish to attain while practicing IF. In certain circumstances, it is not required, but if your objective is to lose some weight, you should still keep track of your calorie consumption.

Also, if you decide to skip snacks before bedtime or stay without eating for an extended length of time, your calorie count will automatically decrease. Another thing to keep in mind is that eating largely plant-based meals will automatically reduce your calorie consumption.

- **Should Women Approach IF in a Different Way?**

In most situations, men and women react to the IF regimen differently. Most women also think that extending their eating window helps them get greater outcomes. When attempting to adopt the 16/8 IF plan, for example, some women found that modifying the method — raising the duration of eating hours to 10 or lowering the fasting hours to 14 - improved their outcomes.

Experiment and see which one works best for you since this is sound advice. Pay attention to your body's indications and indications. Also, see how it responds to a certain IF pattern. Maintain a strategy that seems to elicit good and pleasant reactions from your body.

- **Is Fasting Safe for Women Who Are Pregnant or Breastfeeding?**

For pregnant women, IF is not suggested. It is because your priority throughout pregnancy should be to provide your body with vitamins that will support your health as well as your baby's growth and development. You must consume meals that are rich in nutrients that will aid in the development and growth of your child's body and brain.

Long fasting periods should be avoided if you are nursing. It is due to your baby's ongoing desire for nourishing milk. Fasting can have a significant influence on the quality or supply of breast milk, so be cautious. If you are nursing, it's a good idea to prevent fasting for longer than 12-14 hours to ensure that your milk supply isn't disrupted.

Make sure to keep an eye on yourself and your body. If you discover that your milk production has abruptly dried up and you believe it is because of IF, you should immediately cease fasting. To see whether eating more often fixes the problem, try it. If you discover that fasting is affecting your milk supply, it may be wise to stop for a bit and resume after you have stopped nursing.

- **Is it possible to exercise when doing IF?**

Yes, you certainly can. If your fasting duration is longer than 24 hours, you should plan your exercises on non-fasting days to make sure that you have the stamina to finish them. Other ladies may be seen working out even while they are fasting, particularly if their fast is short than 24 hours.

It is because they have seen how efficient fasting-induced exercise is for gaining lean muscle mass. In general, one should plan your workouts depending on how the body behaves and your previous training routines.

Bonus: 21-Day Flexible Meal Plan to Burn Fat

Prepare to put your 21-day plan into action; it will be critical in putting you on the road to success with IF. But it is not all or nothing. Each week is different and tailored precisely to the dishes in this book. Within the plans, you may alter or change meals. Keep in mind, however, that the nutrients for each daily meal have been determined and are available in Chapter 9. As a consequence, matching the macronutrient makeup of the meals you are changing will provide the greatest outcomes.

• Week 1

This week's low-carb diet plan will keep insulin levels low, allowing for constant fat burning. This diet is ideal for people who are a novice to low-carb diets and love a wide range of animals and plants meals.

Weekly schedule	Meal 1 (Breakfast)	Meal 2 (Lunch)	Meal 3 (Dinner)
Day 1	Apple Cinnamon Oatmeal	Grilled Green Goodness Salad	Sheet Pan Steak

Day 2	Strawberry Shortcake Yogurt Bowls	Chicken Drumsticks Wrapped in Bacon	Filet Mignon Salad
Day 3	Blueberry Lime Almond Muffins	Butter Chicken	Roasted Cauliflower Rice
Day 4	Herb Scramble with Spicy Tomatoes and Mushrooms	Greek Chickpea Waffles	Banana And Cacao Pudding
Day 5	Tomato Baked Eggs	Chicken And Broccoli Caesar Salad	Spaghetti Bolognese
Day 6	Ham Omelet	Almond Thyme Green Beans	Chicken Burgers
Day 7	Vanilla Cinnamon Pancakes	Curried Chicken Salad	Baked Scallops

• Week 2

This meal plan's meals keep carbohydrates to a minimum, allowing your body to enter ketosis and maximum fat burning. This diet is ideal for anybody who struggles to lose weight while yet enjoying robust meals.

Weekly schedule	Meal 1 (Breakfast)	Meal 2 (Lunch)	Meal 3 (Dinner)
Day 1	Salmon And Kale Frittata	Grilled Green Goodness Salad	Red Chicken Curry with Zucchini Noodles
Day 2	Herb Scramble with Spicy Tomatoes and Mushrooms	Filet Mignon Salad	One-Pan Prosciutto-wrapped Shrimp and Broccoli
Day 3	Veggie Omelet	Curried Chicken Salad	Pork Lettuce Wraps with Spicy Cucumber Salad

Day 4	Apple Cinnamon Oatmeal	Chicken Ranch Chop Salad	Salmon And Kale Frittata
Day 5	Herb Scramble with Spicy Tomatoes and Mushrooms	Greek Chickpea Waffles	One-Pan Prosciutto-wrapped Shrimp and Broccoli
Day 6	Blueberry Lime Almond Muffins	Creamy Mushroom Soup	Lamb Patties
Day 7	Veggie Omelet	Banana And Cacao Pudding	Spinach And Feta-Stuffed Chicken Breasts

• Week 3

This week's menu offers a variety of nutritious-low carb dairy and vegetable items to keep your body fit and your stomach satisfied while also helping you lose weight.

Weekly schedule	Meal 1 (Breakfast)	Meal 2 (Lunch)	Meal 3 (Dinner)
Day 1	Veggie Omelet	Filet Mignon Salad	Spinach And Feta-Stuffed Chicken Breasts
Day 2	Cranberry Chutney with low-fat Toast	Healthy Chia and Oats Smoothie	Greek Meatballs with Chunky Tomato Sauce
Day 3	Tomato Baked Eggs	Greek Chickpea Waffles	Red Chicken Curry with Zucchini Noodles
Day 4	Apple Cinnamon Oatmeal	Almond Thyme Green Beans	Grilled Green Goodness Salad

Day 5	Berry Prune Juice Smoothie	Filet Mignon Salad	One-Pan Prosciutto-wrapped Shrimp and Broccoli
Day 6	Veggie Omelet	Mustard Rosemary Brussels Sprouts	Cauliflower Pizza Crust
Day 7	Banana And Cacao Pudding	Curried Chicken Salad	Spinach And Feta-Stuffed Chicken Breasts

Conclusion

Women's health may face new obstacles when they enter their 50s, such as a slowed metabolism, difficulty to lose weight, excess belly fat, stiff joints, and decreased muscular strength, making it difficult to stick to a rigorous diet plan. However, the reality remains that everyone wants to appear slim, lose weight, and feel good.

The good news is that intermittent fasting (IF), a versatile health plan that aids weight reduction and much more, is available. Intermittent fasting also has a long-range of possible health advantages.

If you wish to burn fat, reduce weight, and stay in healthier condition, IF is a terrific alternative. This diet is about more than just the things you consume. It is all about when you consume these meals so that you may stay healthy and have your body perform the heavy lifting for you.

The most difficult aspect of this plan is teaching oneself not to eat constantly. We have been told that eating low-calorie, low-carb foods would help us lose weight, but this is not true for everyone. You may obtain the results you want without having to fight as hard if you use intermittent fasting.

Intermittent fasting is more than a weight-loss strategy. It aspires to be something greater. It provides a number of health advantages that will help you lose weight while also keeping you healthy and disease-free. While looking good is rewarding in and of itself, the significance of improving the duration and richness of your life cannot be underestimated.

So, if you are tempted by old habits or a desire, grab a light snack and study the motivational ideas we have given, go for a nice walk, or call a buddy to accompany you for 1 of your planned pleasures. Remembering why you are doing what you are doing and appreciating how you look, and feel might help you get over any roadblocks on your route to improved health.

Recipe Index

Thank You

Thank you very much for taking the time to read this book. I hope it positively impacts your life in ways you cannot even imagine.

If you have a minute to spare, I would really appreciate a few words on the site where you bought it.

Honest feedbacks help readers find the right book for their needs!

Louisa Perry

Made in the USA
Coppell, TX
30 August 2021

61488442R00105